All My Patients Have Tales

ALSO BY JEFF WELLS

A Veterinarian's Handbook for Horse Husbands

All My Patients Have Tales

Favorite Stories from a Vet's Practice

Jeff Wells, DVM

St. Martin's Griffin ⚔ New York

www.stmartins.com

Book design by Ruth Lee-Mui

The Library of Congress has cataloged the hardcover edition as follows:

Wells, Jeff, D.V.M.
    All my patients have tales : favorite stories from a vet's practice / Jeff
Wells. — 1st ed.
        p. cm.
    ISBN 978-0-312-53739-5
    1. Veterinarians—Anecdotes. I. Title.
SF745.W46 2009
636.089092—dc22

                                                        2008035868

ISBN 978-0-312-60639-8 (trade paperback)

D 10 9 8 7

In Memory of My Father

Contents

Acknowledgments

A special thanks to all the folks who made this book possible and helped along the way: Mary Anne Mier, Rebecca Finkle, Jenny Hancey, Jenny Ramsey, and Mike Daniels.

All My Patients Have Tales

Feline Frenzy

Mrs. Perkins was methodically explaining the symptoms that her new cat, Henry, was experiencing. Although she hadn't had him long enough to know him well, she said it was obvious he wasn't feeling up to par. Mrs. Perkins was a vibrant blonde in her early thirties, with the typical Norwegian Dakota accent. Her husband traveled a lot for his job, and she was elated to have a fuzzy new companion.

She looked me up and down skeptically, clearly evaluating the new guy on the block. I had been out of veterinary school for only a few months. I'm sure it was more apparent than I would have wanted to admit that I was still a little nervous about every case that walked through the door, afraid that I might not be able to handle the situation or that I might misdiagnose the ailment of a beloved pet.

"I just picked him up from the Humane Society two days ago and he was fine then, don'tcha know," Mrs. Perkins began. "Then last night, he began to howl when he went to use the litter box. It was the most horrible noise I have ever heard a kitty make. You've just got to help him."

Even though I was a novice, I had a pretty good idea what was afflicting the recently adopted feline. "Do you know why he ended up at the Humane Society, Mrs. Perkins?"

She pondered for a moment before responding. "You betcha, I remember now—they said he was urinating on the owners' carpet the last couple weeks."

These were the classic signs of a urinary infection, and the howling indicated that a bladder stone was now blocking Henry's urethra, making it nearly impossible for him to empty his bladder. I would need to palpate the bladder to see how full it was and take an X ray to determine the exact location of the blockage. Henry was still in the blue plastic carrier that Mrs. Perkins brought him in. I set it on the Formica exam table between us.

I opened the metal-grate door and began to ease my hand in to get hold of the patient. My hand was almost to the cat's head when his new owner remembered an important piece of information. "Oh, Doctor, I almost forgot—Henry is practically feral. You can't pet him or pick him up. I had to coax him into the carrier with food and slam the door." This was definitely information I could have used earlier! Now I stood frozen, with my arm elbow-deep in the cage of an uncivil feline. On instinct, my hand began to pull back, but it was too late. A sharp pain shot up my arm, and the familiar sensation of warm blood washed over my palm. Henry had sunk his teeth into my index finger.

A white furry tornado then spun out the door of the carrier, tearing at my forearm as it made an escape. Henry hit the floor at a dead run and slid on the linoleum tile as he rounded the corner, disappearing through the doorway of the exam room. Still in shock from my own injuries, I bent over, holding my damaged limb against my abdomen, and held back words that would be unacceptable in rural South Dakota. Mrs. Perkins began to tear up. "Oh, Henry! Please don't let him get hurt or escape outdoors," she pleaded. "He's so fragile."

This statement brought me back to my senses and I began to imagine how upset Mrs. Perkins would be if Henry did manage to make it outside or got hurt trying. I took off after the frightened feline, temporarily forgetting my shredded hand.

Henry had made it into the reception area and immediately started climbing the curtains. Determined to bolt, he seemed to have reached a maximum level of hysteria, spewing excrement randomly as he scurried from drape to drape. The question I frantically pondered was how to get hold of the frightened cat without exciting him even more or losing a limb in the process. While I stood in the middle of the room, wondering why this situation had never been described to me in veterinary school, he made a full circle by using the curtain rods as a trapeze set, then disappeared into the next room.

Mrs. Perkins yelped as Henry streaked by her in the hallway and made for the laboratory, the one room with the most potential for damage by an overstimulated kitty. Following the trail of rancid diarrhea and wondering how the intestinal tract of just one ten-pound cat could possibly produce so much, I followed him into the lab. By this point, I felt sure that Henry was displaying some as-yet-undiscovered biologic mechanism that generated an infinite amount of fecal material, because it now blanketed the once-pristine countertops and sterile instruments in the room. The only good news was that he had decided to take a hiatus behind the autoclave and was now peering out at me from behind it. His pupils were wide open with fear, and the backs of his eyes reflected the fluorescent lighting, giving them a greenish yellow glow. He sat still as a statue, like young deer or rabbits when approached in the deep grass, seeming to believe, If I don't move, the human won't see me.

Now I had to decide how I could get hold of Henry without making the room even more of a disaster zone. For lack of a more brilliant plan, I turned to the basics. "Kitty, kitty, kitty," I called, trying to sound as loving as possible under the circumstances. It didn't work. These words only seemed to alert the frozen feline that I could actually see him, jolting him back into action across the countertop. "Oh, no, not those!" I hollered, but it was too late. The thirty-plus blood tubes that we had worked so hard to get from the unwilling two-hundred-pound pigs the previous afternoon crashed to the floor with just a little shove from Henry. It had taken hours to extract the blood for viral testing. My inexperience, combined with the determination of the hefty swine, had provided a year's worth of entertainment for the farmer and his neighbors. Now I would have to call him, explain the situation, and endure the ridicule of another trip to the farm. I could already picture the scene: Even more locals would be invited this time. Chairs would probably be set up and maybe even tickets sold. But first, I still had to retrieve this cat.

I decided then that I had had enough. Henry made for the door to exit the lab, but I stood my ground. This time, he hesitated, giving me that crucial split second. I dived and scooped him up, keeping his glistening white teeth at bay. He wiggled and clawed at me, making his way up my shoulder. Then he abruptly stopped moving and appeared to relax. He was hanging by one paw from my earlobe. The razor-sharp claws had punctured the fleshy portion of my ear deeply enough to support his weight. I don't know if he had finally given up from exhaustion or had just decided to claim victory, but it seemed that someone had turned off his switch.

When Mrs. Perkins found us, her reaction was not what I might have wished. Instead of saying, "I'm so sorry. Are you okay, Doctor?" she said, "Oh, you haven't injured my Henry, have you?"

With the feline still attached to my ear, blood running down my neck, and Mrs. Perkins scolding me about proper pet restraint, I began to reflect on what exactly had brought me to this point. Eight years of strenuous college curriculum, national board exams, and a huge student-loan debt all added up to this glamorous title of veterinarian, which I had coveted for most of my life.

I wondered what my friends from college were doing now. Probably sitting in plush offices, making big bucks, and working with clients who didn't regularly bite them, I guessed. Yet I really do enjoy this sometimes crazy career choice of mine, and I can't imagine not having chosen it, even though I'm not always appreciated by owner or patient.

Removing Henry from my ear, I carried him back into the exam room, where the whole fiasco had begun. Once he was on the table, he continued to appear relaxed and fairly normal. Mrs. Perkins held on to him while I slipped a sedative into his rear leg. I don't know if he felt better or was just out of fight, but he put up with me. The sedative took over in a few minutes, allowing me to pass a urinary catheter to relieve any blockage. He went home with antibiotics and a change of diet to help prevent any recurrence.

So why did I decide to become a veterinarian? It isn't an easy path; it requires years of hard work just to get that D.V.M. degree and the diploma to hang on a wall, followed by long hours for moderate compensation once you've got a wall to hang it on. To explain myself, I think I'd better start from the beginning.

How You Get There

At least once a week, I am presented with a young boy or girl who wishes to become a veterinarian. These kids' parents are often standing proudly behind them, faces beaming. These future vets always have a great love for animals and a deep sense of dedication. But I have to choke back the urge to awaken them to the long, arduous training and all-nighters that lie ahead of them before they will actually be able to heal an animal. Usually, I just summon a smile and pat them on the head, wishing them the best of luck. I always visualize a little of myself in these eager faces, which reminds me of why I longed to become a veterinarian and what got me through those eight years of college.

To understand what led me down this wild road, we have to flash back to my childhood. I grew up in a small farming community in southeastern Iowa. On the edge of the Bible Belt, it was not a big tourist destination, but it sure was a great place to be a kid. It's still the kind of place where most everyone knows everybody else and people really do take care of one another. Retail shops surrounded a picturesque town square with a bandstand in the center. Weekly instrumental concerts filled steamy summer evenings, and towns-people enjoyed the music from the comfort of strategically placed lawn chairs. It was a town that might have inspired Norman Rock-well, and it hasn't changed all that much in the last forty years.

We lived on a small "hobby farm" just outside of town, where I kept almost every type of pet at one time or another. Cats, dogs, horses, cows, sheep, and even pigs sometimes ended up on our little acreage. Active in the local 4-H club, my sisters and I proudly showed off our menagerie at the county and state fairs in late summer. Fortunately, my father made a living teaching agriculture at the high school, so we didn't have to count on our animals for income like the real farmers.

My favorites in our collection were a Saint Bernard named Heidi and a white Welsh pony named Midge. Heidi and I logged many hours of roughhousing, which usually ended in her pinning my shoulders onto the lush lawn with her front paws, then bathing me in saliva with her immense tongue. This was before canine oral care had gained popularity, a fact that sent me straight for the shower before sitting down for dinner.

Midge spent most days grazing in belly-deep grass pastures, but she always rose to the occasion when she was asked. She could be ridden without a saddle or bridle. You could just jump on her back and take off for a ride across the property, no tack required. Midge was also a big draw on grade-school field trips. Our class would fill up a school bus and head for the petting zoo we called home. Everyone got a ride on Midge, and she was more than happy to oblige. Kids would fall off and even end up underneath her, but she would just stop and wait for them to get back on. These days, of course, insurance companies would never allow such activities for schoolkids.

Growing up around all these animals made it easy for me to answer the age-old question of "What do you want to be when you grow up?" with "A veterinarian, of course." Conveniently, the local veterinary clinic was less than a quarter of a mile from our house. I got a job cleaning kennels at the clinic after school and spent available weekends riding along on farm calls. Soon I was hooked, and there seemed to be no other logical career path.

I'm sure my teachers felt there was no way that I would ever be able to make the grades required to get into veterinary school, but sometimes being told you can't do something makes you even more determined to accomplish it. When it came time to graduate from high school and head for college, I was filled with anticipation. I arrived at Iowa State University determined that, with a little hard work, I could make the cut, but I was in for a big surprise. Reality hit when I opened the new campus phone book soon after I arrived and was completely taken aback by what I saw.

It seemed that almost every other freshman in the university phone book was a prevet student, too. There must have been four thousand of them, and Iowa State's veterinary college accepted only about eighty in-state students every year. My heart fell as I turned the pages and began to wonder what my second choice for a career might be. After a couple hours of couch time spent staring blankly at the television in utter dejection, I mustered the energy to crawl into bed. With the covers pulled over my face, I came to the realization that I had already purchased all the books for my classes, and I'd spent years telling everyone that I wanted to be a veterinarian. So for now, I decided, I at least had to give it a try.

The first couple of years involved lots of chemistry, physics, and many other assorted "weed-out" classes. Many of my fellow students had what seemed to me a truly amazing ability to act like they had everything under control. These people did such a great job of putting on a front that I was certain I was the only one who was struggling, even when using every available minute to study.

Once, after a big physics test during my sophomore year, I noticed a girl standing at the bulletin board, pondering the test scores. I had been looking for an excuse to talk to her for over a year and now took this opportunity to do so. She was very attractive and exuded confidence, making it extra hard to initiate a conversation. "Tough exam. How did you do?" I managed to say while safely staring at the computerized spreadsheet taped to the wall.

There was an uncomfortable silence. I began to assume she had no interest in talking to me, when she breathed a deep sigh and turned toward me. Her eyes were misty, and tears began to spill down her face. In a matter-of-fact tone, she declared, "Well, that's it for me. I've gotten D's on all the exams in this class, and my grade point average can't take it. No veterinary school for me." I was shocked. She had always appeared to be a confident shoo-in, but all was not as it appeared. Concluding that this probably wasn't the best time to ask her out, I walked away, and I never saw her again.

Toward the end of junior year, it was finally time to send in my application for veterinary school. This meant taking the Medical College Admittance Test, the same exam taken by medical school hopefuls. It was one of those exams that actually shorten your lifespan—at least I think it did mine, for the next two days proved to be the longest of my life. Put a few hundred extremely nervous preprofessional students in one lecture hall and you can practically smell the tension. I felt nauseated for most of the forty-eight hours, especially when I realized there were entire pages of questions about which I was completely clueless. This accounted for areas on my answer sheet where the filled-in dots formed an assortment of geometric patterns that I'm fairly sure had nothing to do with the correct answers.

A few months later, the letter from the Iowa State College of Veterinary Medicine appeared in my mail slot. I stood staring at it, wondering if not knowing was better than knowing and being disappointed. Realizing that someday it would have to be opened, I tore into the envelope. "This letter is to inform you that you have . . . not been accepted for next year's freshman class."

I wanted to put it back in the mailbox and ignore the fact that I knew. But it was too late—the genie was out of the bottle, and now I had the terrible task of telling my parents and friends. Everyone else took it better than I did, and even though I wanted to run away and become a ski bum, I decided to give it another try.

I learned later that without a bachelor's degree, getting accepted on the first try was almost impossible for anyone. In fact, several applicants already had master's degrees. A year later, after completing my degree in animal science, the envelope contained a much better answer. It was a day of celebration, and I remained blissfully ignorant of what lay ahead the following fall.

Four years of undergraduate work, during which I was constantly stressed about keeping a high-enough grade point average to be accepted, culminated in my finally arriving at that mythical first day of veterinary school. I sat in the last and top row of the stark freshman lecture hall. The chairs were early-modern plastic, attached to imitation wooden desks barely large enough to hold a piece of notebook paper. The dean was explaining the rules and regulations of the school while the front-row crowd frantically took notes. They were at it already, the same students who had raised the curve in my prevet classes back on the main campus. Which of the dean's general remarks could possibly need to be written down? I wondered. These front-row students were working hard to impress the "right people" early on. As it turned out, these attitudes and seating arrangements would remain the same for the next four years.

The veterinary school was well over a mile from the heart of the university. The building was immense and partly below ground, which is where freshmen were kept for most of their first year. It was constructed of concrete blocks, with just enough windows to remind us what sunlight was like. The stark white walls were interrupted periodically by orange metal doorways and bad seventies art. The school was completely self-contained, everything under one flat roof.

Most of the time, it seemed, we were completely isolated from the rest of the world. In some ways, it was a lot like high school: This school, too, was equipped with locker rooms, and we had our own intramural teams. We would be with these same 120 people for almost half a decade, and some would become lifelong friends. We took all of our classes in the same building, studied there, and occasionally slept there. I think we sometimes forgot we were allowed to leave.

The first day of class in any anatomy lab always brings with it the concern of how one will react to the cadavers. I was fortunate enough to have grown up around life and death in our little farming community, but some of my classmates were not so blessed. A few of the most affected bolted for the rest room, while the rest of us spent most of that first lab class suppressing our gag reflex, trying to maintain an image of coolness in front of our new cohorts and competitors. After a few weeks, dissection became more routine, and we settled into our new adventure.

Freshman year provided us with a continual flow of extremely helpful and devoted professors. Each of them seemed to feel that his particular subject was the one we couldn't live without, no matter how impractical it might be in the real world of veterinary practice. I can still remember the names of a multitude of exotic diseases found only in the most remote areas of Africa.

That inaugural year ended in a flurry of final exams, which pushed each one of us to the limits of his or her mental and physical capacity. I opted to put off studying for my last exam, which happened to be in histology, to concentrate on the other subjects first. Unfortunately, this left me looking at an all-nighter.

The histology final was two hours long, the time spent mostly staring into a microscope. About halfway through, every student's worst nightmare happened to me: I actually fell asleep during the test. My eyeballs pressed against the optics of the microscope. I still have no idea how much time passed during my nap, but when I awoke, a feeling of panic swept over me. Searching the room for a clock through my groggy daze, all I could see were my fellow students busily analyzing the glass slides that had been specifically prepared for the exam. I scrambled to finish evaluating the cells that we had spent the last year fretting over, barely finishing when the professor called time. The little siesta cost me the grade I had hoped for, but at least I hadn't missed the whole thing.

It's been many years since that awful experience, but up until the last couple of years, I would still occasionally wake up in a cold sweat, sure that I had missed my finals altogether or forgotten to go to a specific class for an entire semester. I think of it as my own personal version of post-traumatic stress syndrome.

Our sophomore year was probably the toughest scholastically, but having one year under our belts made it a little easier to adjust. We had also gotten to know one another well enough to know who our friends were and who might be out for themselves only. Classes like pharmacology, microbiology, and virology dominated the scene. You know it's a tough year when crying is a regular occurrence after reading the posted test scores. But we held on, wading through it with the knowledge that junior year would bring more practicality and hands-on experience.

The third year did bring more practicality. We even got to work with animals in some of our classes, such as reproduction lab. Pregnancy diagnosis is an important part of almost every veterinarian's career in both small- and large-animal practice, so this was an important introduction. Unfortunately, with large animals, pregnancy diagnosis always involves a long latex glove. We were dressed in our brand-new white coveralls with smart veterinary emblems sewn on the right-hand chest region. A potentially pregnant cow was placed in front of each student and, one by one, we made our determinations.

The girl beside me was particularly nervous about this task, as she had not been around cattle before that day. She whispered in my ear right before her turn came. "I only want to work on cats and dogs. I really don't care to do this." Eventually, her turn came to give it a try. An extremely large holstein cow was led in front of her while she put on a large latex glove and lubed up her arm. She placed it inside the cow as far as she could. As luck would have it, the patient had spent the last couple of weeks on a particularly lush Iowa pasture and was anything but constipated. By this time, my fellow student had her shoulder actually inside the cow, making the beast a little agitated. Finally, the immense bovine arched her back and directed all the abdominal pressure she could muster to force the student's arm out of her for good.

But my comrade was more determined than one might think, not easily yielding to the cow's wishes. Her arm must have been positioned at just the perfect angle, because an explosive stream of pungent green liquid stool found its target on my classmate's face. She was temporarily transformed into the Creature from the Black Lagoon. We all felt very sorry for her, but she was able to laugh about it after a couple of weeks of utter humiliation.

Our senior year was split between the clinics at the school and working in actual veterinary practices. We came and went from the school to the "real world" and back again. During our time at the school, we saw patients before our professors did, trying to make the correct diagnoses while still under experienced supervision.

As school began to wind down, we all started to think of leaving what was still at least a somewhat sheltered academic world. Most of us had put in at least eight tough years preparing for practice, but now that we were almost ready, it seemed like a scary prospect. Would we be successful, or would we fail miserably? How could we possibly remember all the information that had been thrown at us over the years? One by one, my fellow classmates started accepting jobs all around the country. We shared many sad good-byes, knowing that most of us would never cross paths again.

This time was hard for me and also made me nervous, inciting a desperate interviewing blitz. I looked at jobs from California to Maine but couldn't quite find the right fit. I had imagined myself leaving the Midwest, yet when a very intriguing offer came in from eastern South Dakota, I couldn't pass it up. The location didn't sound very glamorous, but I really liked the veterinarian who owned the practice, and the facilities were first-rate.

I decided to accept the position and packed up my red 1973 Mercury Marquis with all my belongings. I had no idea what I was in for.

Baptism: Reality Strikes Back

I arrived at the clinic the next morning to start the first day of work, meet the staff, and begin to learn the ropes. Pulling into the driveway at 7:45 in an attempt to make a good impression, I saw that the main structure was a split-level, with offices in the lower level and living quarters on the upper floor. Directly to the west of the converted house, about thirty feet away, sat a fifty-foot-square one-story barn with stalls for keeping sick horses and a surgery area that included a hydraulic operating table for large animals.

I found the facility still fairly quiet, with the steamy haze of a midwestern morning just starting to blow off. My new employer said a quick hello as he passed, heading out to a full morning of farm calls, leaving me awkwardly trying to find something to do. I walked into the main building and gave myself a tour. The waiting room and reception area lay straight ahead, and the lab was to the right. The small-animal surgery room, exam room, and doctors' office were to the left. The entire floor in each area was covered with the same yellow linoleum, badly scuffed from heavy boot traffic. The familiar smell of B vitamins filled the place; every veterinary clinic I've been in has smelled exactly the same way. Moving into the office area, I took a seat at what would be my desk. It had recently been cleaned out and was now completely barren, like a clean slate.

The outside door swung open just as I was contemplating what I might use to start filling up my inherited space. Through the door walked a woman who was about twenty-six years old. She had a medium build, was five five, and had shoulder length thick dark hair. She wore a light blue lab coat, gray overalls, and sturdy brown leather work boots—not worthy of the cover of *Vogue* but a good practical outfit for veterinary practice. I stood up to introduce myself, and she began to look me over. Her eyes narrowed and her nose wrinkled. She was sizing me up, and I wondered how I was going to make out.

"Nice to meet you. I'm Jeff," I said, sticking out my hand.

She grasped it firmly, asserting her authority. "You must be the new guy," she replied with what seemed a tinge of disappointment in her voice. "I'm Jenny, your technician, and we'll be spending a lot of time together." What I was sure she was really thinking was, Oh, boy, now I have to train this guy. She dropped my hand and spoke again "You won't actually be treating anything for the first month; you'll be working with the veterinarian whom you'll be replacing."

Ugh, a direct kick to the groin, leaving me with a pit in my stomach and no air left in my lungs. She was good—well versed in putting young veterinarians in their place! Did she not understand the years I had spent preparing for this day? The sacrifices I had made? All-nighters at the vet school, running IV fluids into vomiting dogs, and sucking down caffeine while the professors slept peacefully in their beds? She didn't seem to have any appreciation for the hundreds of tests I had taken or the hours of preparation they required.

Yet, after I got my wind back, I realized that it would probably be a good idea to get some on-the-job training. Besides, I could learn my way around the practice and get to know the clients. So I gave Jenny an accepting nod, and she took off to start her morning routine. This would not really be my first day of practice after all, but that day would come soon enough.

My first real day of practice as a licensed veterinarian was full of a little anticipation and a whole lot of fear. After eight years of preparation, it was finally "go time."

I spent my first month at the practice with the veterinarian I was replacing, meeting the clients and trying to learn as much from her as possible. She was a highly respected veterinarian and possessed an abundance of patience, which was fortunate for me. Dr. Ann had grown up in South Dakota and understood how to deal with the locals. She was barely over five feet tall but was in great shape, so even the most physical task did not appear to slow her down. Her hair was dark, wavy, and always kept short for easy maintenance, a logical style for a woman with such a messy occupation. The clients adored her, as did I.

Jewelry might easily get caught in the hair of a dog or the tail of a cow, so Dr. Ann never wore it. She was personable, honest, and a very good practitioner, but she was leaving this practice to join one closer to her new family, who lived a couple of hours away. She had recently married and had instantly become the mother of two teenage daughters. Obviously, she had her work cut out for her. Dr. Ann would be sorely missed, and I understood that filling her shoes was going to be hard, even with my big feet.

I learned an awful lot from her in that month and became a little too comfortable in my role as her apprentice. Like most young graduates from professional school, I thought that I had at last gained all the knowledge I needed to jump right into practice and save the world from disease and pestilence. As you can guess, I was in for a rude awakening. By the time my month of training with Dr. Ann was up, I was dying to get out there and give it a shot on my own. I figured that my employer, Dr. Dave, would always be there for guidance in my upcoming adventures. On her last day, Dr. Ann shook my hand and wished me luck with a knowing smile. She was all too aware of the challenges ahead of me in the months to come. The next morning, I would be on my own.

I didn't sleep very well that night, trying to imagine myself in a multitude of situations that might occur the next day. I even tried counting sheep, but one of them ended up with a birthing problem that I couldn't remember how to deal with. At last, morning came, and I hurried to get to the clinic early to see what my first tasks would be. This was the last day that I was ever early. I tried to appear casual as I strolled over to the reception desk to glance at my schedule. It would begin with pregnancy testing on horses, followed by a dog spay and an afternoon kept open to catch whatever emergencies might arise. This sounded good, but I knew my afternoon was open because no one wanted to see the new guy. The people of eastern South Dakota did not accept change quickly. I would be under the community microscope for quite some time.

I headed out to the practice truck that I was taking over from Ann, shoved the seat back so I wouldn't be eating my knees, and jumped in. Jenny crawled in beside me, and we started off the day I had so long anticipated. I peered through a kaleidoscope of glass—a windshield beaten by the South Dakota wind and too many gravel roads. The dashboard was stuffed with old receipts, syringe cases, and the occasional candy wrapper. The seats were warped and threadbare, and the smell of antiseptic soaps and vitamins permeated the cab of the truck.

Pulling into the Weber farm, I was a little nervous, yet very excited about being the person they had hired to determine whether or not their mares were pregnant. I approached the house, passing a decomposing truck, rows of barbed wire, and leaning sheds. As at all agricultural operations in the heartland, this one had the obligatory four- to six-foot border of perfectly shorn grass along the drive, an orderly perimeter, defending the homestead from the ever-encroaching chaos of a livestock operation.

The Webers were a tough farm family. They worked very hard to make a living with a herd of about thirty prize quarter horse mares, plus countless numbers of dairy cows and pigs. Mrs. Weber worked just as hard as her husband did, hooking the cows up to the milking machines and keeping the equipment clean. She was a small woman with salt-and-pepper hair. There was not an inch of body fat on her, a result of running miles around the farm while looking after her husband and the animals. Since both of their sons had left the farm to pursue careers that were more financially rewarding, they had to hire part-time help to plant and harvest the crops.

Like most farmers in the area, the Webers lived on the economic edge, so having their broodmares pregnant was very important. If the mares were bred, they could go out to the far pastures; if not, they would need to spend more time with the stallion. Sometimes those that were "open," or not with foal, would even require medical treatment before they could hold a pregnancy. Mares that did not have foals the following spring would not help the Webers' financial situation. The pressure was on me to make the correct diagnoses, and the Webers were big fans of my predecessor, so this was my test run.

I slipped on the long latex palpation glove, without which I would never have been able to get my fingernails clean again. Jenny held a gallon jug, from which she dumped a large glob of gelatinous lubricating jelly into my hand. The first mare stood ready in front of me, restrained in a palpation stock for her safety and mine. I eased my well-prepared hand into her rectum, feeling for the uterus that lay below. I had done this many times before in school or under the supervision of an experienced vet, but this time was different. Instead of easily finding the uterus as before, I couldn't find it or the hard head of an equine fetus. Everything inside the animal felt like unrecognizable mush. I was taking too much time, and the Webers were starting to fidget. Even the horse began flashing me dirty looks. My stomach started to churn while I fought back the urge just to make a break for the truck and run.

Finally, since I could not locate the uterus, I astounded myself by loudly announcing that she was pregnant, then prepared for the next mare. Much to my disappointment, the next one felt the same way. I was getting more nervous with each mare, making the process of determining pregnancy even harder. Making the best decisions I could, I worked my way through the dozen mares to be tested that day. I thought I was going to vomit from the feeling of total incompetence when my hand went into the last horse. Finally, the familiar skull of a foal bounced against my palm. I had just started to feel a little better about myself yelling out "Pregnant," when the mare decided to get in the last word. She kicked out her back left leg with lightning speed, and her hoof cracked against my shin so hard, it sounded like a shotgun blast. I reached down and rubbed it; as no bone was sticking out, I knew I could at least get to the truck.

For the first time, a smile crept across Mrs. Weber's face. Such a gesture, I noticed, was completely foreign to her tired face. She had gotten her entertainment for the day and was not going to hide it. In her mind, the old mare had given me an official initiation. I'm sure it was payback for having taken so long. We said our good-byes as I limped back toward the getaway vehicle. I had never been so glad to be leaving a place in my life.

As soon as we had reached a safe distance from the barn, Jenny couldn't take it anymore and turned to me with a smirk on her face. "You had no idea what you were doing back there, did you?" she asked. I flashed her a disappointed glance. "Was it that obvious?" Jenny rolled her eyes and nodded her head. That was answer enough. Not a stellar start to the inaugural day.

My next job was a dog spay. How tough could that be? I had performed several of these in veterinary school, so I sat up straight again and guided our vehicle toward the clinic with renewed confidence.

On arrival at the clinic, Jenny converted the exam room into a surgery area while I examined the patient. She was a one-year-old Doberman pinscher, Ellie, who appeared to be in perfect health. We lifted her onto the table, and Jenny held off the cephalic vein on the smooth front leg while I injected the anesthetic into it. Like most Dobermans, Ellie sat stoically, not even wincing as the needle penetrated her skin. When she drifted off, we placed the endotracheal tube and hooked her up to the isoflurane gas. Jenny clipped the hair away from Ellie's midline and sterilized the area with Betadine soap.

After donning gloves and a surgical mask, I opened the sterile surgery pack, eventually finding a scalpel, to which I attached a sharp new blade. Standing over the sleeping dog, I made the incisions through the skin and muscle with relative ease, then began the inevitable search for the tiny ovaries. Finding them gave me a little feeling of relief; the first steps were over. Next the ovaries were ligated with thin blue suture material, followed by the body of the uterus, just in front of the cervix.

This is the point in any surgery when you hold your breath, cutting loose the tissue to remove the body of the uterus and ovaries, hoping the ligatures will hold. I slowly removed the reproductive tract from the dog, then frantically searched her abdomen for pools of blood. It looked good—just a very small amount of hemorrhage, which you would expect to see after any abdominal surgery.

I began to close the incision, when a trickle of bright red blood appeared. I stopped suturing and watched it run down onto the green paper drapes that helped to keep the surgery area clean. The flow began to increase, and when I pushed down slightly on the surgery site, blood poured out onto the table and then covered my shoes. It was official: We had a bleeder! As the blood leaked out of the dog, the last bit of confidence drained from me, as well.

For a moment, I froze. My stomach churned and I thought I would vomit all over Jenny. A feeling of loneliness swept over me as I realized I had no professor or more experienced practitioner to turn to. The cold hand of isolation gripped me.

Finally, I realized that in order to save this animal, I would have to do something very soon. With hands quivering, I removed the sutures already placed and dug back into the abdomen to hunt down the bleeder. Bright red blood was everywhere, and Jenny helped me soak it up with four-by-four gauze sponges. Several times, I had to bring myself back from the brink of panic, but I eventually found that the blood was oozing from the stumps of both ovaries. I had double-ligated both of them, and the sutures were holding tight, but blood still welled up from the severed vessels. We proceeded to tie off both sides with more suture material and held our breath. I could see the relief in Jenny's eyes when no new blood appeared. We had before us, at long last, a bloodless abdomen.

I stitched up the abdominal muscle, followed by the subcutaneous layer and finally the skin. This is just what we had been taught in school, but I couldn't help worrying how things were going inside the dog's abdomen. Were my ligatures still holding, or had the bleeding resumed? These are concerns that keep rookie veterinarians up at night.

Jenny removed the endotracheal tube while I was closing, and the patient began to wake up quickly after the last suture was placed. She seemed a little sluggish and pale, so we decided to give her a little extra blood. If I could have, I would have given my own blood, but since that wasn't feasible, we would have to look for a more realistic donor. Just outside the clinic, I found Bud, the resident black Lab. He sat down at my feet, wagging his tail and smiling up at me. It was almost as if he was volunteering.

Fortunately, blood typing is not required for canine blood transfusions if the recipient has never received donor blood before. We pulled a few large syringes of blood from Bud and mixed it with some anticoagulant to keep it from clotting before getting it into Ellie. I injected the life-giving fluid into our anemic Doberman through the IV catheter that Jenny had already placed. Almost immediately, Ellie seemed to perk up, and the pounding in my head began to fade away. Jenny, Bud, and I kept a close eye on Ellie for the next couple of hours. Her gums remained pink, and by about four o'clock, she began to become interested in food again.

I felt very lucky that we all survived that episode, but I was never really sure why she had bled so much. Occasionally, Dobermans can develop a bleeding disorder very similar to that of human hemophiliacs, but the owners declined testing for this condition. We never knew for sure whether the hectic episode was due to a bleeding disorder or just to the inexperience of a young veterinarian.

My first day had proved worse than your average hazing, and just when I thought it was over, the phone rang. One of our hobby-farmer clients just north of town had a cow that had aborted and hadn't cleanly expelled the placenta yet. This, I could definitely handle. Removing the placenta from a cow is usually a fairly straightforward task and doesn't require a whole lot of time. Dave was still out vaccinating some horses, so I knew he would be happy if I could take care of this one. Jenny had had a hard day working with me, so I told her to go on home and said that I would be fine.

When I arrived at the Thomas farm, the cow was already in a holding chute, and a small crowd of observers had started to assemble in the open-sided shed beside her. Mr. Thomas worked at the local meatpacking plant and raised cattle on the side to supplement his income. He was a tall, slender, sort of sad-looking man, about retirement age. His neighbors, for the most part, led very similar lives, and I knew they were not gathering this evening to "shoot the bull." It was time to judge the new vet in town.

I grabbed the long latex sleeves out of the truck, then headed for the business end of the cow. I grabbed her tail and moved it to the side to begin the placental extraction. My heart sank. Besides the expected placental tissues, a small lifeless foot protruded from the cow. Worse yet, the entire area was covered with—oh, yes—maggots! I began to gag a little but then suppressed the urge, as this would be seen as a sign of weakness, which a young veterinarian could not afford to show.

This meant I was going to need a whole new game plan. Mr. Thomas now realized that the calf had not aborted after all, and he was staring down at his feet while kicking the dirt. He finally drew in a long breath to speak. "I'm sure sorry about this; you know, I really thought that calf was already out," he said in his strong Dakota accent. Then he went back to examining his shoes.

I headed for the truck to reequip for a much bigger and more time-consuming task. I rifled through the truck, finally coming up with a pair of calf-pulling chains and a "calf jack" to help me extract what was left of the calf from its ailing mother. This piece of equipment is basically a long pole with a flat bar on one end that fits around the butt of the cow. On the pole is a lever with a pulley and a cable that, when attached to the small chains placed around the calf's legs, is used to wrench the calf from the cow. I proceeded to set up this apparatus without any help from the audience.

Once the chains were in place and the cable hooked on, I began cranking the lever. Eventually, the cable tightened to the point of snapping, but the calf did not budge. I even tried forcing a half gallon of lubricant between the calf and the vaginal wall to help it slide out, but the move was futile. The dead calf had bloated up over the last couple of days and was now stuck like a cork. Still there were no helpful volunteers from among the jurors. The noise level of the conversation was increasing, but most of the onlookers seemed to be ignoring me. I convinced myself that they were just afraid of maggots crawling up their sleeves, but in reality I think they were more like Romans in the coliseum and I was the gladiator.

Nearly an hour had passed since my arrival, and I knew that I had at least that much longer to go before winning this battle. I went back to the truck and came up with some fetotomy wire, a thin metal fiber covered with barbs for cutting apart a dead calf within a cow for easier removal. Although this procedure might seem crude, I knew the cow would die if the decaying calf was not extracted. I delved back into my job with renewed purpose, certain that I could extract the calf this time. But as the clock ticked by and none of the calf had been extracted from the cow, my enthusiasm started to wane.

Meanwhile, the spectators had started to regain interest in my strife. The conversation had almost come to a complete halt, except for the occasional snide remarks about the amount of time that had passed since my arrival. There was beginning to be a lot of head shaking and disgusted looks. Another hour passed, and I finally had to face the fact that the calf was not coming out this way, either. With my head hung in defeat, I turned to Mr. Thomas and sheepishly admitted, "I can't get it out this way; I'm going to have to do a cesarean section."

At that point, a hush fell over the audience and a small figure wiggled to the front of the crowd. The tiny creature with a wizened face approached me. He was about eighty-five, with a worn John Deere cap pulled down over his eyes. He used a cane to support himself, since he was severely bent over at the waist from years of hard farmwork. He looked up at me, raised the cane, and stuck the end of it an inch away from my chest. From under the cap, a voice croaked, "That's what you should've done to begin with!" The end of the cane slammed to the ground and the accuser spun around, disappearing back into the crowd.

So there I was, two hours into a job that should have been done two days before, and now I was being told how to do it. Turning my back to the consenting nods, I went back to work once more. Within the hour, the cow was free of the calf and I was closing the incision. The spectators had dispersed, except for Mr. Thomas, who thanked me for all my efforts, then headed back toward the house, muttering about how long it had taken.

Once I arrived back at my apartment, the brand-new coveralls purchased for my first day went straight into the Dumpster outside. The muscles in my college-boy hands ached from wrist to fingernails, and I couldn't seem to stand up completely straight. I was asleep before the couch knew what hit it. The day that had seemed like it would never come was over. I hadn't saved the world after all—just gotten a little beat up by it.

You Are What You Eat

Puppies are always cute and lovable, no matter what breed, color, or size they are. They are made this way so that someone will inevitably want to take them home. It's nature's built-in puppy-marketing plan. But under that adorable fuzzy disguise can be a little monster waiting to wreak havoc. All puppies will chew on shoes and ruin socks, but occasionally you run into one who carries puppy mischief just a little too far. Often these puppies seem to mistake rocks, wood, or even sanitary napkins for dog food. These diets almost always lead to vomiting and diarrhea, always on the best white carpet in the house. It was these symptoms that led to a concerned phone call on a steamy Dakota morning in late August.

The receptionist relayed the message that Mr. Ramsey had called in to say that his new Border collie puppy, Sam, was not doing well and that he needed to bring him in as soon as possible. I had just given the pup his first vaccinations the week before, and Mr. Ramsey was sure that these shots had caused the current illness. It is not uncommon for owners to blame their pet's current problem on the animal's most recent veterinary procedure. More than one phone call from a client has begun with the person saying, "You saw my dog two years ago, and now he's very sick," insinuating that whatever I did then directly caused the completely unrelated sickness now affecting the animal. I told Mr. Ramsey to bring Sam in and said that we would get to him as soon as we could.

It seemed as if I had barely gotten off the phone when Mr. Ramsey burst through the door, even though he lived ten miles away. He held an exhausted-looking Sam in his thick forearms. Even though he was seventy-four years old, Mr. Ramsey's body had not yet given in to time. He wasn't a tall man, but he had the wide wrists and the huge hands of a man who had carved out a living for half a century on the northern plains. He had recently retired from farming, but he still wore the uniform of his trade: a white T-shirt under a pair of blue denim bib overalls with the waist buttons undone in case there was a big midwestern meal coming up. As with most farmers who have dealt with livestock all their lives, Mr. Ramsey tried to act like the puppy didn't mean that much to him. "I wasn't that concerned about him—he's just a dog, after all—but . . . the missus talked me into bringing him in." This macho image was paper-thin; the concern in his creased face gave him away as he gently placed the emaciated puppy on the exam table. He explained that Sam had vomited a couple of times in the middle of the night, but he was sure the pup hadn't eaten anything out of the ordinary.

Upon examination of the puppy, all I could find abnormal was some hard stool in the posterior abdomen. Since everything else turned up normal, I concluded that the little guy was just constipated, and we all know how bad that can make you feel. After injecting some electrolyte solution under his skin to keep him hydrated, I sent Sam home with some laxative tablets. Mr. Ramsey seemed happy with this treatment and thanked me heartily as he tucked Sam under his big arm to head for home. Unfortunately, I didn't share his exuberance. I had a feeling we were not out of the woods yet.

I spent the afternoon vaccinating a group of especially unappreciative young horses that required my undivided attention, realizing only at the very end of the day that we still had not heard any more about Sam. Right before the clinic closed, I called in on my truck radio to see if Mr. Ramsey had made contact. I caught the receptionist just before she made her 4:59 P.M. mad dash for the door. She informed me that in no way, shape, or form had Mr. Ramsey been in touch with the clinic that afternoon, and then cut me off, as if I was about to ruin her entire evening. I smiled as I imagined her stomping out and slamming the door at 5:01 P.M.

All evening, I kept thinking about the little dog, hoping he was not getting any worse. I even had a dream that a very upset Mr. Ramsey had called in the middle of the night to tell me that Sam had died and he was going to sue me for malpractice. It was one of those nightmares when you have to sit up and look around the room for a while before you realize it was just a dream. I actually had to check in with the answering service before convincing myself that no one had paged me.

After a night of less-than-perfect sleep, I couldn't stand it any longer. The minute eight o'clock rolled around, I called the Ramseys to check on Sam's condition Mrs. Ramsey was quick to tell me that it hadn't changed a bit. I told her that we had better get the little guy in for some tests. If she could just drop him off for the day, I said, that would be best. She protested about leaving him at first, but after I convinced her we would not perform any "scientific experiments" on

Sam while he was with us, she promised to get him in. Apparently, as Mr. Ramsey explained to us later, she had recently watched an investigative special on television about the cosmetics industry's use of animals for laboratory testing.

That day, we performed a barium study of the puppy's digestive tract. This procedure involves administering a little sedative before passing a tube through the animal's mouth into the stomach, then inserting a liquid through the tubing that will show up as white on an X ray. Next, Jenny and I took several well-timed radiographs as the barium moved through the intestinal tract. The X rays revealed the classic signs of blockage where the barium stopped in the large intestine and would not move past the large barrier. The mass appeared to take up the entire back half of the dog. My first thought, after examining the radiographs, was that I was just glad they weren't of my abdomen. But I was stumped, unable to decipher what made up the mass. Most often, these blockages are fairly distinct on X rays. Common intestinal plugs in puppies, such as rocks, socks, and children's toys, can be fun to pick out on film. But this monster was definitely something new to me. I showed it to my boss to get a second opinion, but he just scrunched up his face as if he were trying to pass the object himself, shook his head, and moved on to his next case.

Now I would have to come up with some sort of plan on my own. I knew what needed to be done next; I just couldn't face it. Then Jenny said it: enema. Now that she had said it, I would have to perform one. As I stood holding the container of soapy water with the plastic tubing attached, which was now inserted into Sam's you-know-where, I felt so proud, thinking of how I had spent eight years in college to become Dr. Enema. Jenny was holding the little dog's head, trying to hold back what was either a laugh or a dry heave. Finally, after several attempts at breaking up the unrelenting obstruction, I announced that allowing the effect of the soapy water to work its magic overnight would be the way to go, and Jenny called the Ramseys to come pick up their.pup. Surgery would be a big risk for this emaciated puppy, so we decided to give the laxatives and enema one more chance to work.

I was hoping we would get a call the following morning that the concretelike substance was in the middle of their living room floor, but no such call came. I had to look at a horse with a bellyache at a farm near the Ramseys' place, so I decided to stop in and check on Sam. Stopping in to check on a patient unannounced is always a little risky because of the possibility that the owners have taken the pet to another veterinarian or, much worse, the animal has passed away. In this situation, I had to brush off these concerns before turning the truck down the Ramseys' mile-long driveway. I drove through the fields of six-foot cornstalks, which formed a wall of formidable green on each side of the driveway. A yellow haze of pollen hung in front of the car, released from the tassels atop each plant. These fields were no longer planted by Mr. Ramsey; he had sold off all of his farm, except for a few acres where the house sat, so that he and his wife could afford to retire.

I pulled up to the modest white farmhouse, which had a huge vegetable garden on one side and a clothesline heavy with overalls and bedsheets on the other. Walking slowly up the old cement steps onto the porch while holding back the urge to turn and run, I pushed the doorbell, then waited. I had hoped to hear a healthy barking puppy scampering toward the door, but instead the only noise was the creaking of the porch swing beside me.

Eventually, the heavy sound of work boots moved slowly toward the door. Mr. Ramsey stood in the doorway, shaking his head and making a gesture with his arm for me to come in. His facial expression gave me a clue to the situation; I was sure that little Sam was no longer. We continued into the dark living room, where Mrs. Ramsey was kneeling over a fluffy dog bed, her face red from crying. She was embarrassed to be caught showing so much emotion and quickly wiped her tears with her apron when she saw me come in. I started to express my sympathy for their loss, then realized that Sam was still alive. But it was obvious that his condition was worsening. Mrs. Ramsey spoke up. "We really appreciate all you've tried to do for him, but is there anything else we can try?"

I could not believe that the blockage had not passed yet, so I scooped up Sam and headed back to the clinic. I had one more chance to save their little companion. Speeding back out the driveway with little Sam on the seat beside me, I noticed the barrage of grasshoppers smashing against my windshield. It was one of the cyclic years in the Midwest, when the grasshopper population was very high, and my increased speed had decreased their ability to clear out of my path. On the route to the clinic, I thought again about the curiosity of puppies and began to develop a theory.

Back in the treatment area, Jenny and I fired up the enema apparatus again with renewed hope. Once the tube was inside the dog, it was obvious the laxatives had begun to do some good; the blockage had moved back quite a bit. We continued to flush in the fluid, and eventually a couple pieces of the blockage broke loose. Just as I had surmised on my trip back to the clinic with Sam, out came grasshopper legs! Sam had not been able to resist the bouncing, brightly colored insects and felt it was his job to rid the world of all of them. We continued to break down the mass with the enema fluid, and a continuous flow of grasshopper parts emerged. By then, we were both beginning to feel a little nauseated as the stench of decaying insects filled the room.

After an hour of continual work, the last of the "Grasshopperlith" was removed, and within another hour Sam was feeling a lot better. Jenny offered him a small dog treat, which he gobbled right down. I called the elated Ramseys and told them they could pick up their little friend, but I suggested they might want to keep him inside until the grasshopper blight was over.

Mr. Ramsey soon appeared to get the pup and thanked us profusely while receiving a thorough face cleansing from the unobstructed canine. Alleviating constipation will make anyone ecstatic. Mr. Ramsey happily paid his bill, made some little joke about how expensive grasshoppers were, then trotted out the door.

A few weeks later, I drove past the Ramseys' farm on my way to another client's. With the corn gone by then, I could make out in the distance a slightly larger Sam chasing a bright orange butterfly through the manicured yard. I cringed automatically as the worst-possible scenario came to mind. Hopefully, it won't be a big year for butterflies, I thought.

Holiday Pay

A big disappointment to most young veterinarians is the amount of time that is spent being on call for emergencies. Unless the practice is located near a fairly large city with an emergency clinic that will take calls about small-animal problems after hours, carrying a pager is a regular part of life. The weekends and holidays off, duty become a valuable commodity.

The next big surprise is what some clients feel is an emergency. All veterinarians joke about how many times a client will watch a sick or injured animal for days, only to call it in as an emergency on Sunday afternoon. And once the client has made this decision of urgency, the vet must deal with it immediately!

One of these situations happened to me on a lazy Labor Day weekend early in my career. I was enjoying a sunny afternoon jog on a quiet Dakota back road when my electronic leash went off. Stopping at a pay phone next to a gas station, I learned John Erickson had a lame draft horse stallion on his farm west of town, about an hour away. I told him that we would be glad to see him first thing Tuesday morning. But he replied quickly, "Ah, Doc, I was hoping you could see him today. He's been sore for about a week, don'tcha know." I gave it one more shot. "It will cost more to see him today than tomorrow," I told him, but this didn't slow down Mr. Erickson.

Reluctantly, I ran back home, checked my truck to be sure the right equipment was accounted for, and headed off. The route to the farm passed by dozens of family picnics in front of big old white farmhouses with wraparound porches, yards perfectly manicured and littered with red, white, and blue. Such picnics are an aspect of America that is too often left behind for amusement parks and megamalls these days. Such family get-togethers are something I still miss about rural life.

After about an hour, I pulled in the driveway I was looking for and turned off the engine. Like the other farmsteads, it was well groomed and a flag was flying. In fact, the barn and house were in even better shape than most, but there were no picnics in this yard. Mr. Erickson was standing by the big red barn, waving for me to pull the truck over closer to him. He was a tall, friendly man, sporting the typical striped overalls and required seed-corn cap. He greeted me with a big smile and a handshake that took me a few minutes to recover from. He had the hands of a man who was not afraid of hard physical labor, even at an age when most men would have been retired. "I appreciate your coming today," he mumbled, then slapped me on the back hard enough to leave me speechless.

We headed in to see Big Mac, the delicate flower John was so concerned about. He had a sore right rear foot all right, but at 2,200 pounds, he was a little more than I was willing to grab hold of and start poking around. We decided that a little sedative might be helpful. After all, I would be working on the business end of the horse, and it was easy to imagine him drop-kicking me through the barn wall. After an injection of sedative into the monstrous animal's garden hose–diameter jugular vein, his formidable head began to drop and the pain in the hoof was temporarily forgotten. Fortunately, he was a gentle giant, and with the assistance of the tranquilizer, he let me examine him without objection.

I worked quickly, trying to find a sore spot on the hoof, while John patiently looked over my shoulder. Time was of the essence, since the sedation would last only about twenty minutes. Finally, I found a spot in the hoof that made the big boy withdraw his leg slightly. With my hoof knife, I dug into the tender area, and white pus oozed out onto the old plank floor. A pungent rotting odor immediately followed, but Mac was going to feel better very soon. Once the pressure in an abscess is released, pain relief isn't far behind. After wrapping the foot with gauze and duct tape (yes, it works on animals, too!), I gave him a big injection of long-acting antibiotic just before the sedation began wearing off.

John started to become a little more talkative now that his draft horse was going to be okay. We struck up a conversation while waiting for the last of Mac's hangover to dissipate. He began to tell me how his wife had died a few years before, after a bout with cancer, and his children had moved away in search of better jobs. His daughter lived with her family in Chicago, and his son in North Carolina, where he had a career in computers. You could see his disappointment that neither had stayed home to run the farm, but he understood it was a tough way to make a living in today's world.

He told me about how his parents had emigrated from Sweden and were part of a Swedish settlement near the farm. John had attended a one-room schoolhouse, where classes were taught in both

English and Swedish. We talked way past the time it took for Mac to wake up. He told me about his life on the farm and how it was interrupted only by the time he spent in Europe during World War II. We talked until the shadows began to get long and Mac began whinnying to get back with his mares.

John finally said, "Well, it's probably time you want to go?" I responded that I had probably better get back, and he nodded with a disappointed understanding. I waved good-bye and headed for home just as the sun tucked itself in behind the rows of tasseled corn. The yards were now getting dark and the people had moved inside. Only the multicolored glow of televisions could be seen through the old four-pane windows.

I never saw John again, but I have thought about him often. He was from an era when we were more of an agricultural nation, when children inherited the farms and the necessary skills to run them from their parents. That period was in sharp contrast to the modern-day one, with its large mechanized corporate farms, which require only a few people to work thousands of acres.

It was sad to consider that the sun was also setting on the family farm and John's way of life. After originally having been upset about being dragged out on that holiday weekend, I realized it was a gift to be able to spend time with this man and his horse.

Always Take Clean Clothes

 Although I have never been a big-time cattle practitioner, some of the bovine calls have provided me with the most entertaining experiences of my career, and a call I got one January day was definitely among those. The middle of January in eastern South Dakota is not ideal for a veterinarian who does any large-animal work. Needless to say, it was extremely cold—so cold, in fact, that the trees and bushes were encased in a white frost just from the moisture in the air. It was like driving through an enchanted forest made of fine crystal—beautiful, but so frigid that just breathing froze the hairs in your nose.

I swung my Ford 150 pickup into the clinic driveway, hoping to have an easy morning and be able to spend most of it performing small-animal surgery in the well-heated surgical room. Alas, I was greeted by the receptionist, who informed me the Schmidt family had a cow that was having trouble calving. My heart sank. Fortunately,

Jenny, my technician, had also just arrived, so we scooped up the appropriate equipment and headed for the truck. Jenny was quite grateful that the truck was already warmed up, and she hopped right in. The full blast of the heater kept the frost off our bodies but warmed up our boots just enough to remind us of what we had stepped in the day before.

The Schmidts were a couple in their thirties who owned a little farm on the edge of town. They raised a small herd of Simmental cows and would have been considered hobby farmers in most agricultural circles. They both had jobs in town, so they ran the farm in their off-hours.

The heat in the truck was beginning to put me to sleep, and I almost missed the driveway. But the Dakota air knocked the sleep right out of me when I opened the door of the pickup. Jenny and I were prepared for the weather in our traditional South Dakota garb: Carhartt overalls, stocking caps, and snow-ready boots. It wasn't exactly fashion-runway material, yet we knew it would come in handy that day.

Mrs. Schmidt greeted us, drinking a steaming cup of coffee and holding a bundled baby on her hip. "They're out there"—she pointed—"but we don't have a catch pen or a head gate."

This was not good. While I've always respected people's right to own livestock, there's nothing more frustrating than needing to treat an animal and not having the proper equipment to restrain them. Chasing an upset bovine with a half-born calf in subzero weather was not the way I had hoped to spend the day.

We saw our problem standing in the far end of the pasture with two forelegs hanging from her backside. "Do you think you could rope her?" Mrs. Schmidt asked. Oh, why did she have to bring that up? I was terrible with a lasso, and now I would have to give it a shot. Retrieving my rope from the truck, I explained to Mrs. Schmidt that

I was not skilled enough with a rope to catch the cow, but I knew an attempt would be necessary to prove it to her.

Meanwhile, Jenny had made her way across the field and was moving the patient back in our direction. As the cow ran by, I tossed the lariat in her general direction. To all of our surprise, she literally stuck her head in the loop as she dashed by. But my jubilation quickly faded when I realized that now I had a fifteen-hundred-pound animal on the end of a rope. She realized it, too, and bolted off, with me holding on for dear life. With her assistance, I was suddenly taking six-foot strides, practically flying through the air. The scene must have looked like something from an old Road Runner cartoon. I was determined not to let go, in order to try to save the calf. I knew catching the poor cow again would be practically impossible. This went on for a good ten minutes, with me sailing behind her like a rag doll on a string.

Between gasps, I yelled for Jenny, pleading with her to try to chase the cow toward one of the big corner posts on the outer fence. But rather than come running as she usually did, Jenny stood in the middle of the pasture, not moving. She just stood there like a statue even when I continued to yell for help.

At last, the cow slowed and I was able to tie her off to one of the posts. After taking a moment to catch my breath, I slipped the calf chains around the greasy forelegs hanging from the cow and pulled with all my remaining adrenaline. Much to my surprise, the calf was still alive. His head and tongue were swollen, yet his legs began to move when I pulled. Just when I thought that I had nothing left, the glistening little fellow slid out onto the ground. Within five minutes, he had shaken himself off and found his mother's udder.

Human newborns are so helpless and completely dependent on their mothers. But animals just born have no time for rest, as a predator could be lurking just around the corner. A bellyful of fat, rich milk and off they go. I am still in awe every time I witness a birth. So many things have to go perfectly for months to achieve a living, breathing being. I'm not sure how well Darwin's theory stands up to this kind of perfection.

I gathered my equipment, my hands now aching from the cold, and put it back in the truck, again with no help from Jenny. She just stood beside the vehicle, looking forlorn. I climbed into the cab and started it up. Jenny slowly opened the passenger door but didn't get in. She wouldn't even look at me and just stared at the ground. I couldn't hold back any longer. "What were you doing back there? I really needed your help," I told her bluntly.

Still no response, but I watched a tear roll partially down her cheek before freezing. Finally, she spoke softly. "I'm sorry I didn't help, but I was laughing so hard watching you run behind that cow, I . . . I wet my pants." Then she turned around. The seat of her coveralls was completely soaked and starting to freeze. She had been totally paralyzed with embarrassment! How could I be upset with her now?

I covered her side of the cab with old surgical towels from behind the seat and gave her a reassuring smile. We took off, heading back into the frosty Dakota landscape, laughing about the whole crazy experience.

Watchdogs?

I had learned growing up in rural Iowa to be wary of what might be protecting the farms and the occupants within. Usually one or more mixed-breed dogs would come running from all corners of the barnyard to converge on me when I'd visit somebody else's farm. Most achieved satisfaction just from striking fear in my heart and would commence wagging their tails as soon as their mission was accomplished. But others took themselves a little more seriously. Tough dogs come in all different shapes, sizes, and breeds. Just because a dog looks like a kind old retriever, I've learned, the rules may change when it comes to protecting his domain.

Size can also be deceiving. I have walked to many a front door with a Yorkshire terrier attached to my ankle. With tough dogs, I have learned protective tricks, such as holding my hands high on my waist and not making eye contact. Looking an aggressive dog in the eye is usually perceived as an act of war, which ends, for most people, in a mad dash back to the truck.

People's fear of dogs ranges from one end of the spectrum to the other. My own sister is deathly afraid of the canine species. One Christmas break, she and I were shopping for gifts in my hometown when we were approached by an old beagle as we came out of a clothing store. The little dog had obviously birthed more than her share of puppies, as her teats nearly dragged on the sidewalk. She was making the rounds, begging for treats, while her owner was solving the world's problems with his cronies on the town square. At the sight of the big brown eyes and joyful tail wags, my sister dashed back into the store as if she had seen the devil himself. It's hard to believe that we come from the same gene pool.

Normally, dogs are not a big problem when you know what you're getting into. It's when you are visiting a new client and taking that first cautious step out of the truck that things can go awry. On this particular cloudy Dakota afternoon, Jenny and I pulled into the small farm owned by Jim and Sally King. They had owned the place for only about a year and were just getting it cleaned up, as the previous owner had died after a long nursing home stay. They had been in the clinic with a couple of cats that required neutering, but none of us had ever been to their farm. Now we were there to see a foal with a facial laceration.

I stepped cautiously out of the truck and waited for the typical anarchy brought on by my arrival at most farms, but nothing happened. I knew that the Kings would not be home. When they set up the appointment, we were warned that they would be at their day jobs in town. Jenny and I were to treat the foal in the barn, then leave them instructions and a bill on the front door. Unfortunately, they had neglected to let us in on a crucial aspect of their barnyard.

Jenny and I headed toward what at one time could have been called a barn. Now it was more of a lean-to with a couple of stalls and just enough siding left to slow the wind down. One of the stalls contained our young patient and her mother, who was watching over her and eyeing us suspiciously. The little brown filly had a small cut over her right eye, where she had most likely bumped her head while romping in the stall. Jenny grabbed the filly by the tail and the neck so I could inject a small amount of tranquilizer into her jugular vein. Within a minute, the little horse relaxed, and I dropped down on my knees in order to get close enough to the filly's bloody head to clean up the wound. After injecting some lidocaine into the skin around the injury to numb it, I was able to close the wound with four sutures.

Standing back up after half an hour of concentrated work, I found my knees were soaked with the familiar horse urine and feces that have ruined countless pairs of my jeans over the years. (My wife still gets a little frustrated when trying to find a decent pair of pants for me to wear to a social event.) The end result was a success, despite my smelly knees. Except for the fish line–like sutures, it looked as if the wound had never happened. Fortunately, a facial wound usually heals well due to the good vascular supply in that area, so the scar would be very minimal.

Little girls always ask two questions of me when their horse is injured. The first is, "Will my horse be okay?" This is followed quickly by "Will there be a scar?" This young horse owner would be happy with both of my answers. You never know when a small blemish could keep an animal from a blue ribbon at a horse show years down the road. According to little Sara King, this new equine was destined to be a champion show animal.

While we were cleaning up, I was sure I noticed something move past the spaces between the boards on the side of the old barn. I had not forgotten the lack of a canine greeting on our arrival. In fact, I'd had a gut feeling the whole time we were working on the filly that we were not alone. As we started toward the truck, I noticed another movement from behind some bales of hay stacked in the barnyard. This time, Jenny noticed it also, and we agreed the quick motions resembled those of a bird. We were both becoming a little anxious by the time I headed for the front door to leave a note for the Kings. Jenny eased up into the truck cab and closed the door quietly. I got to the entryway, where I left a detailed note and some penicillin to give the filly for the next week.

Turning away from the door, I prepared to make a beeline for the truck, when I realized what had been stalking us. Three full-grown male turkeys were staring me down just five feet away. Normally, turkeys would not be that much of a concern, but these big guys appeared to have a purpose, and it seemed to involve me. Their heads stretched to chest level, their large sharp beaks draped in the customary loose red skin. They reminded me more of prehistoric raptors from a Steven Spielberg movie than next year's Thanksgiving dinner. They remained statuesque until I took that uneasy first step toward the truck. This gave them the green light to attack, and they swarmed around me as if my clothes were made of bird food. I broke into a run, but they cut me off.

The three of them worked as a team, alternating their lunges. Eventually, a sharp beak drew blood from my forearm. Farmers sometimes kept a turkey to protect their sheep from dogs, but this was ridiculous. It was time to up the ante. I picked up a long stick from the ground and began swinging it in front of their ugly red heads, hoping to scare them off. But they were very determined and were not intimidated by my poor excuse for a weapon.

Meanwhile, Jenny was enjoying all the action from the safety of the passenger seat. Slowly, while wielding the stick like a sword, I made my way to the truck and jumped in when Jenny opened the door. I gulped for breath, still clutching the stick in my hands. Jenny continued to roll with laughter until I brought up the fact that the vet box was still open in the rear of the truck. Her face went immediately sober as she began begging me not to make her get out and close it. I eventually gave in, but I knew the box would still have to be closed, or the medications it contained would fall out on the bumpy driveway.

There was no way I was getting out with the killer avian creatures squawking just outside my door. Jenny pointed out that the rear window in the cab had a small sliding window. After a short struggle, I popped through, crawling along the toolbox until I reached the open vet box, the turkeys flying at me all the while in a last attempt to kill their prey. Back in the cab, I fell in behind the wheel, leaving the frustrated birds in the dust like a bad dream.

I didn't mention the incident to the Kings, figuring they already knew what monsters they kept. In fact, Jenny and I were a little too embarrassed to tell anyone right away, but we knew one day we would be called back out to remove the filly's sutures. A few weeks later, the call came in, and I felt anxiety creep over me, as I anticipated a return to Jurassic Park. I asked the receptionist if the Kings had mentioned whether or not they would be present this time and was elated to hear that they would be.

Opening the truck door that next afternoon, I was relieved to see Mr. King waving at me from in front of the barn. We exchanged greetings and I went on immediately to remove the filly's sutures. Jim nodded his approval and made a joke about my bright future in plastic surgery.

I was a little nervous as we walked to the door of the house so Mr. King could write a check for the call. I was having flashbacks from the previous visit and was just about to bring up the killer turkeys, when I saw little Sara standing in the open doorway. She began to thank me for fixing her filly, and it was then that I noticed the red marks covering her face and arms. My jaw must have dropped, because Mr. King felt he needed to explain. "Those darn turkeys got her down in the front yard. It was lucky I was within earshot." He sighed. Before I could ask the obvious question, he went on to say that the big birds had been the guests of honor at the church's last potluck supper the previous Sunday. This information gave me great confidence on my trek back to the truck. The next time we called on the King farm, I was happy to discover that they had a new Labrador puppy guarding the property.

Jailbreak

One of the biggest nightmares in any veterinary clinic is having an animal escape from the facility. Every time an animal makes a break for the outside, my blood pressure goes up as I frantically hope that all the doors and windows are closed. Most clinics have a multitude of measures to prevent this from happening, but in our small-town mixed-animal practice, it wasn't that big a concern—until one pet changed all that.

The local bank president, James Van Meter, had a tough little dog named Bingo. James was the classic banker, with a crisp, clean pinstriped suit, perfectly groomed hair, and a good handshake. His dog was a cross between a Border collie and a German shepherd. Bingo had had a rough start in life, having been dropped off at an animal shelter when he was just a puppy. Sadly, he was the product of two purebred dogs whose owners were embarrassed by the impure offspring, so as quickly as possible, the pups were removed from the premises. But now Bingo was the pride and joy of the Van Meter family. He was fat and sassy, as well cared for as any animal could be. His gray coat shined, and a new leather collar encircled his thick little neck.

Now he was long overdue for a little elective surgery. Men often put off neutering their male dogs. It's a macho thing, I guess; you would think we were going to do it to them.

James dropped him off on a brisk November morning, and we got to him about eleven o'clock. I collected the surgery pack and antiseptics while Jenny went to get the patient out of the kennel. When Jenny reached into the cage to retrieve him, Bingo proceeded to bite her arm. Her initial reflex was to grab the injured limb with the opposite hand, which gave the dog just the opportunity he was looking for. Evidently, he had somehow realized what he was at our office for and had decided against it.

He flew from the room, making the corner just as my boss was coming in from outside. Dr. Dave swung the door open, and the pup didn't miss a stride running through it. Jenny had recovered and would have caught up with him if she hadn't slipped on the linoleum. The dog blew out the door, passing Dr. Dave and heading for town, which was just a couple of miles away. Bingo was on a mission. He stretched out to cover the maximum amount of ground with each stride, causing his body to become closer to the ground, like a cheetah on the hunt. His ears were flat against his head to minimize wind resistance, and his tongue hung out to the side, flapping in the breeze.

Jenny and I were panic-stricken. We started to follow on foot, but Bingo had a head start and there was no way that we were going to catch him that way. The thought of Bingo showing up at the bank, still in possession of the parts we were supposed to remove, made me cringe. Even worse, he might get hit by a car on the road.

We looked around for something to help us capture him. Then we noticed an old fishing net hanging on the wall of the clinic garage. I had found it just a few days before on the highway, where it had probably fallen from someone's pickup. It had a four-foot handle and a diameter just wide enough to get around Bingo. The netting wasn't in very good shape; part of it was torn too much to hold a fish, but I hoped not enough for a canine to slip through. I grabbed it and we jumped in the truck. The chase was on.

Jenny was driving and I was riding shotgun with the fishing net. By the time we were out of the driveway, she had the truck up to thirty miles per hour and was throwing gravel and dust. She was pushing forty when we spotted Bingo in the distance, running flat out. He was in the ditch beside the road, making a beeline for home. Going fifty miles per hour, we were finally catching up with him.

Jenny pulled alongside Bingo, who was still at a dead run and did not appear affected by our presence. Bingo didn't even look up at us as he concentrated on his goal. Jenny pulled just ahead of the dog and hit the brakes. I grabbed the net and jumped from the truck. By the time I gained my footing, Bingo blew by in the tall, dry prairie grass. I made a feeble attempt with the net, but it was way too late. Within seconds, I could no longer see the escapee, just the grass parting as he ran ahead of me.

Fortunately, Jenny was thinking more quickly than I was and pulled the truck about a city block ahead of our prey this time. She barely got the vehicle stopped on the shoulder before jumping out and disappearing into the sea of brown vegetation. By some miracle, it came to me what she was up to, so I started running in the direction of Jenny and the dog. I'm sure the scene of me running crouched like a Masai warrior with an old fishing net for a weapon would have made for quite a laugh down at the coffee shop. Suddenly, Jenny jumped up right in front of Bingo. He paused, stunned by her appearance, then turned in my direction. The look of disappointment on his face when he saw me just a few feet from him was undeniable. Had he been capable of speech, I'm sure his reaction would not have been repeatable in public. He tried to dodge to the left, but I was pumped up on adrenaline by then. With a last chance leap of desperation, I went for it. It was one of those times when you feel like you're in slow motion. I closed my eyes and hoped for the best. When I opened my eyes, the dog was already biting at the fishing net from the inside in a last-ditch effort to regain his freedom.

Relief flowed into us as we drove Bingo back to the clinic to complete the task that we had started. I was not about to take our less-than-happy captive out of the net for the ride back. He just sat on my lap and growled occasionally, attempting to bite me.

Back at the clinic, an anxious Dr. Dave awaited our victorious arrival. His scowling face lighted up with a broad smile when he saw the netted pooch. I'm sure he had been debating whether or not to call the liability company. This time, we turned the building into Alcatraz until it was time for Bingo to go home. When James came to pick up his pet, he was completely oblivious. He even commented on how good Bingo looked after having been through an operation. Evidently, no one had seen our little comedy routine, so we all decided to let sleeping dogs . . . Well, you know how it goes.

Was It Something I Said?

A few nights before my first Christmas in practice, the pager went off about 6:30 P.M as I was getting ready for a date. I groaned at the realization that I would probably not be going on the date after all, and dates had been few and far between for me recently. The answering service said that Dan Meyer had called in from north of town. His daughter's horse had been caught in the barbed wire and was bleeding badly. The date was definitely off at that point.

Dan was a nice guy, just a few years older than I was at the time, with a young family. But that night, he didn't have the best timing. After yanking off my dress shirt, I picked up the phone and called to cancel the date. The young woman tried to act as if she understood, but she was not a big animal lover and I knew it would be the last time we would talk. So, instead of dinner and a movie, it was out into a South Dakota snowstorm.

Turning the key in the ignition of my pickup, I heard the engine groan against the cold, turning over very slowly. I pressed the pedal to the floor on the second try, and the engine roared to life. I had no time to let it warm up because the horse was bleeding badly. As I rolled out onto the interstate, the wind pounded against the truck, forcing me to keep the steering wheel turned into it. At times, the gusts were so strong that it was hard just keeping the tires on the pavement. The worst part was that no one else seemed to be on the road, creating a lonely, almost eerie feeling on the interstate. No one would find me tonight if I went off the road, I told myself morosely. They were all in restaurants or movie theaters, or cuddled in their homes, smart enough to stay out of this weather.

Finally, the exit appeared and a narrow gravel road led me to the Meyer farm. Pulling in the driveway, I could see the old farmhouse illuminated by the beam from my headlights. It was badly in need of paint and a new porch. Beside it was the barn, or what was left of it—a skeleton of its former self. The century-old roof had fallen to the ground on one side, and a soft light came from the section that was still standing. Knowing that was where I would find the patient, I made my way through the snow toward the light.

The plan was to evaluate the situation before dragging out my weapons of choice. Inside the dusty barn stood the little mare, blood-soaked old rags wrapped around her lower right front leg. Beside the horse stood Haley, the young owner. Eyes swollen, tears frozen to her face, she looked up at me as if I were the grim reaper. Someone had already prepared her for the worst. Behind me, her father stumbled in out of the storm and shook off the snow. Pulling off his cap, he bellowed out, "Well, Doc, what do you think? Can you save her?" It was the kind of question that always makes me cringe, and it did so especially that night, since I knew I would be held to my response by young Haley. Explaining that I had not been able to take a good look yet, I proceeded to take off the saturated bandage.

Haley watched with great anticipation as the bandage slowly came off. The dried, frozen blood had solidified the rags into something that resembled a plaster cast. When I finally wedged the last of the rags loose from the leg, blood began to flow freely again. There was about a six-inch cut with a pumping artery in the middle, but no tendons or joints had been damaged. Turning toward Haley, I smiled and winked to let her know the mare would be okay. "She'll be good as new before you know it," I announced. "But it's going to take some sewing tonight and lots of rebandaging on your part." Father and daughter both smiled, acknowledging that they could handle it.

After a couple of trips to the truck for water, suture material, and bandages, the task of putting things back together began. I ligated the big bleeder and carefully closed the laceration, knowing that a minimal scar was going to be a big deal later on. Meanwhile, Haley and her dad reminisced about the ribbons that she had won at the county horse show the previous summer. Finally, I finished bandaging the leg, and they helped me carry the equipment back to the truck. As I was cleaning up the instruments, they headed for the house. Haley's dad yelled for me to come on in so we could "settle up."

Inside the modest kitchen, a steaming cup of hot chocolate waited on the table, and the whole family watched as I sipped it while writing up their bill. Almost forgetting that I had been pulled away from my date, I felt my frustration wane with the warm cocoa in my stomach and the sight of Haley's new baby sister asleep in her crib next to the heating vent.

Looking down the narrow hallway, I noticed that some of the rooms were temporarily closed off so they wouldn't have to be heated. As I sat there with the young family, scribbling down the charges, I found myself leaving out a few of the items. The total ended up significantly less than it should have, but things were obviously a little tight in this household. Haley's mom wrote me a check and stuffed a Tupperware container full of warm chocolate brownies into my hand.

The truck started right up this time, and I looked in the rearview mirror, to see Haley waving from the lighted doorway. I was feeling pretty good about having that call behind me and thinking about heading for a little TV, then bed, when the unthinkable happened: The pager went off again. Since we were not equipped with cell phones yet, I pulled off at the next exit and ran into Lucky's Truck Stop. I spotted the row of pay phones they had for the truckers to use, found a vacant one, and called the answering service. A client had called about her cat, who was not using the litter box. I was telling her what to do until she could get in the next morning when I noticed that the trucker on the phone beside me was acting a little strange.

He was a tough-looking man with a lot of tattoos and a big bushy beard, and he must have tipped the scales about a biscuit shy of three hundred pounds. His dark, wide-open eyes seemed to be focused completely on me, but instead of anger, they were full of fear. He slowly put down the phone and started to back away as if he had seen a ghost. Then he turned away and practically ran out the door. I looked all around me but could not figure out what he might have been so afraid of. No one else was close by. Eventually, I looked down at my hands. They were covered with dried horse blood from the tips of my fingers to my elbows. I had forgotten to wash off after suturing Haley's mare. The poor man probably still believes that I had just committed mass murder, but I wonder whom he thought I was talking to on the phone.

Under the Big Top

Many times in life, things come up that sound like a lot more fun than they really are. One day, we received a call at our clinic that the animals with the traveling circus, which had been performing in town for the last week, needed blood tests and health certificates to travel into Canada. After hearing this call come in, my employer took off in his truck for what was to be a "full day of farm stops," leaving me to do what I thought would be a lot of fun. Jenny and I loaded the truck with extra blood-collection tubes and headed for the fairgrounds, where the circus was set up. She was just as excited as I was. "I always wanted to get up close to the animals at the circus," she said, eyes dancing. But I wondered if it wasn't the muscle-bound, shirtless acrobat men whom she really wanted to see.

We began to realize what we were in for when we pulled in behind the big top and no one was there to greet us. I guess we expected a welcoming committee. Egos slightly deflated, we began looking for someone to help us with the procedures, or at least to point us toward the animals we were to test. As we walked around the grounds looking for Hans, who had originally set up the appointment, we started sensing that the circus workers were not overly happy to see us. When we asked them where we could find Hans, they just grunted at us like New Yorkers reacting to a tourist with a map. They obviously didn't really want us there. I expect they felt that their privacy was being invaded by what probably seemed to be forced testing of their animals. As I thought about it, I realized that they had probably had veterinarians discover problems in the past that had kept them from moving on to their next destination.

Finally, after confronting at least a dozen circus folk, we found Hans, a Fabio look-alike who appeared to be in charge of all the four- and two-legged animals. His impressive stature and chiseled face demanded respect not only from employees but also from us. He looked us up and down with an expression of disappointment. Then, after an uncomfortably long stare, he finally spoke. " 'Bout time you showed up. Try not to dillydally, and I want the paperwork done ASAP so we can move north!" He pointed out the locations of the animals that we were to examine and strode off to his more important responsibilities.

The next thing I knew, I was trying to get blood from a full-grown elephant. At no time during veterinary school had anyone mentioned how to go about finding a vein on an elephant. It seemed like something one might want to do right the first time, while inflicting minimal pain. One of the handlers finally pointed out that a previous veterinarian had gotten blood from the vein in the rear leg, but he seemed to derive great amusement from my lack of knowledge before giving me this hint. The approach seemed to be satisfactory with the elephants, so we went with it and made our way down the row of giants standing in knee-deep fresh yellow straw. I breathed a sigh of relief when the last syringe of pachyderm blood was full and Jenny had gently packed the tubes away. Breaking one of these sample tubes would mean coming back for more, and the patients might be a little more agitated with us the second time around.

Next we moved on to checking the camels for tuberculosis. After injecting all four of them with test material, I was able to walk away with only one faceful of camel spit. We then examined the horses for any sign of contagious disease, relieved by now to see an animal we were used to dealing with. The beautiful white equine entertainers showed no abnormalities, but there was still one group of animals that I had put off until the bitter end: the big cats! They had five African lions and twenty-one tigers that needed to be checked over. I realized that I would not be listening to their hearts with my stethoscope or examining their gums for ulcers. The question was, How close did I really need to get to these man-eating felines in order to feel like I was still doing my job? The kitties were all in their individual cages, lined up in three rows—except for one, which was positioned a significant distance away from the others.

The guardian of these cats was a tough-looking sixty-plus woman sitting on a stool, legs crossed, in front of the first row of cages. She had a small thin brown cigar hanging from her mouth and glared at me through the curling smoke that framed her face. She grunted at me in her thick Eastern-bloc accent, "Don't get too close; you will upset them, and they have a long reach." Then she trailed off, grumbling in words that were not English but were probably not complimentary, either.

I now knew why my boss had run from the circus adventure. Trying not to show too much fear, I proceeded to bend over and peer into each cat's lair without stirring the animal up too much. Jenny hung back. "I'll start the paperwork," she whispered.

Yeah, right, I thought, but at least she could call 911. Most of the big cats just lay calmly in their cages, while a few others growled playfully or even rolled over on their backs. I hurried down the rows and was relieved to be nearly finished when I headed for the last one in the back.

The keeper of the cats snarled something unrecognizable at me again and shook her head slowly. I later realized that she was trying to tell me, Don't go near that one. The big tiger got one look at me and slammed his body against the cage door, pushing the limits of the latch and hinges. He let out a bloodcurdling roar and tore at me through the bars. I leaped backward, falling into the cages behind me and thus upsetting the rest of the cats.

By the time I gathered myself back together and made sure my bodily functions had held, the big top felt more like a bad day on the Serengeti. I tried to leave quickly, with a tiny bit of dignity left, but the last of it was drowned out by the hearty laughter of the tiger lady.

After enjoying Jenny's account of the day in the safety of the clinic, my employer volunteered to deliver the final test results and paperwork the next day. He just couldn't bring himself to make me go back there, no matter how funny the story might have been if I'd had to return for a second round.

Second Opinion

An old veterinarian told me when I first became interested in veterinary medicine, "Veterinary practice is five percent what you know and ninety-five percent dealing with people." This was hard information to swallow for an aspiring veterinarian who expected that scientific information would carry him through any situation in practice. Most veterinarians, myself included, enter the field for the classic reason—because we love to work with animals. This is great, but it might be better if we could learn from the time we were kids to think, I want to become a veterinarian because I love to work with animals and their owners. Some of the most successful practitioners I have known had not only good clinical and surgical abilities but also great people skills.

I learned the hard way how valuable the ability to work well with humans can be early in my career in South Dakota. A horse client of mine called about four o'clock one afternoon to see if I could help her out with a "sticky situation." A horse that was boarded at her farm was having some problems standing up, and the lady who owned the horse normally used another veterinarian. The problem was that the other vet had been called out four hours earlier but had not arrived yet. When I asked who the other vet was, the voice on the other end of the phone hesitated. "It's Doc Bob," she said finally. Doc Bob was almost a legend in the area. He was seventy-five years old and had practiced in the region his entire career. Most of the locals loved him, but younger veterinarians tended not to be big fans. He was very hard on new graduates and felt that only he was qualified to treat the local animals.

My client, Mrs. Hoye, was getting worried that the horse might die before Doc Bob arrived, so she begged me to come out and take a look. With much regret, I headed out to check on the poor animal, praying that I wouldn't run into Doc Bob in the process. I let Jenny stay back at the clinic, since it was so late in the day and she had indicated that she might have some plans for the evening.

The Hoyes' stable was about ten miles away from the clinic, and I tried to make it as quick a trip as possible, hoping to get there and back before the old veterinarian showed up. I pulled into the driveway, which looked down onto the vast pasture below. In the middle of the field, the horse lay on its side, and standing over the poor animal was the stooped figure of old Doc Bob. Mrs. Hoye ran up to the truck to meet me. She was a tall, attractive woman in her midforties. She had a kind smile, which didn't fit with the cigarette that always hung from the corner of her mouth. "I am so sorry. He just arrived," she said quietly, as if she was ashamed to have bothered me now that the long-awaited "master" had arrived. I was just relieved that I hadn't been the one who had arrived first and started to examine the animal, only to be brushed aside by my esteemed colleague.

I said my good-byes to Mrs. Hoye and began to back down the driveway, when I spotted a short little arm motioning to me from the pasture. This was exactly what I was trying to avoid. Doc Bob was motioning me down to assist him. My plan to escape unnoticed had failed, and now I was stuck. I realized that if I continued to pull away, it would be considered rude, and I would appear not to care about the ailing horse. If I stayed, I risked being made a fool of by the experienced gray-haired practitioner. Why else would he be sucking me into this situation except to teach me a lesson? I wondered. Surely he had seen hundreds of similar cases before; besides, he was known to be an expert in all veterinary matters.

After reparking the truck, I shuffled reluctantly toward the recumbent horse to take my lesson in humility. Doc Bob was in the middle of explaining the reasons that he was certain the animal was afflicted with snakeroot poisoning. As he ranted on, I scanned the pasture for the white flowers characteristic of snakeroot that time of year. I would have found his diagnosis easier to swallow if there had been any of these plants in the field, but I was not about to interject that thought at this point. After the dissertation was finished, he announced that it would be best if the animal was put down immediately.

By now, Jamie Marshall, the patient's owner, was cradling the comatose horse's head in her lap and sobbing inconsolably. A young woman in her mid-twenties with big brown eyes, messy black hair, and a face that was swollen from crying, she managed to interrupt her grief just long enough to say, "I don't want to lose him. Isn't there anything else we can do?" Her dark eyes begged as she looked to the old veterinarian for a glint of hope. Now I was wishing that I could turn and run, because I knew what was coming next. But for the sake of the animal, I couldn't leave. Then Doc Bob actually acknowledged my existence. He looked at me coldly and asked the fatal question, "What do you think?" Mentioning my name would have given me too much credibility, when all he wanted was for me to agree with his diagnosis and treatment.

I just stood there, trying to pick my words carefully. Mrs. Hoye caught my attention; by raising her eyebrows, she hoped to encourage a second opinion. Searching for just the right words, I pointed to the two-inch cut above the horse's right eye and replied quietly, "What do you think about that?" I hoped to appear as humble as possible in insinuating that a blow to the head might have initiated the neurological symptoms.

Doc Bob scowled at me; obviously, he had expected that a greenhorn would not dare to disagree with him. He quickly dismissed the injury as having occurred after the snakeroot had taken effect. Yet Miss Marshall wanted desperately to try some kind of treatment, and after my thoughts were out in the open, Doc Bob could not turn back. He snapped at me, "So how would you treat him?" His impatience was becoming more apparent as he glanced back and forth between his watch and me, realizing that his supper was going to have to be microwaved.

I suggested the usual head-injury treatment of corticosteroids and IV DMSO (a common antiinflammatory for animals). He turned up his nose at the mention of DMSO. In his words, "It makes everything smell like a garlic factory." Besides, it would take at least an hour to run in through an IV catheter. He stared me down as if I were the Antichrist, sent specifically to ruin his day.

Finally, the silence was interrupted by Miss Marshall's hopeful voice. "Can we try it, please?" she asked. Since it was his patient and I felt I had done enough to irritate him, I said my good-byes and made tracks for the truck. A great wave of relief began to rush over me as I felt almost ready to distance myself from this uncomfortable case.

My hand was almost on the door when I sensed that someone was on my heels. It was easy to imagine jumping in the pickup and burning rubber to escape, but I could not ignore the incessant throat clearing from Doc Bob just behind me. "What dosage of those drugs would you use?" came out as if he were giving me a test. After giving him the appropriate doses, I watched as he rooted though his truck, hesitating to analyze an occasional bottle in hopes it would be the correct one. About ten minutes of this frantic searching had elapsed when I decided to retrieve the medications out of my truck, then handed them to him. He scowled at me one more time, then scurried off toward the patient, clutching my supplies as he went.

Mrs. Hoye thanked me profusely for coming out, especially since Doc Bob had gotten there after all. "It's no problem." I grinned, and behind my smile was elation. Escape from this call without Doc Bob publicly embarrassing me was all I could ask for.

The next morning, I arrived at the clinic, wondering how the horse had fared. Within five minutes of walking through the door, Mrs. Hoye was on the phone to update me. Miss Marshall was riding the horse back to her own house as we spoke, and he was doing great! It made me happy to know that the horse would be fine, yet I couldn't help but wonder how the owner perceived the legendary veterinarian now. It seemed obvious that he had slipped off his pedestal at least for a moment. I have to admit that it gave me a warm feeling to think that I might be perceived as less of an amateur by those who were present, but I was in for a surprise.

Having let the incident slip to the back of my mind and having moved on with life, the whole thing came rushing back one morning a couple of months later. I had stopped to get gas at one of the local convenience stores and I noticed Miss Marshall coming out the door. Playing dumb, I asked her what had happened to her horse that evening. She looked me up and down with a tinge of disgust on her face. "Well, he's doing just fine. Hasn't missed a beat since you saw him last." Her eyes narrowed as her face moved closer to mine. Then she spoke in an almost lecturing tone: "That Doc Bob, he's a miracle worker. The absolute best. You could learn a few things from him."

It was at this point that I really understood why Doc Bob had such a viable practice: He could convince people of anything. It took me a few minutes to gather myself together and get back in the truck. As I drove off, I couldn't stop thinking about the fact that Miss Marshall had been present for the whole conversation between Doc Bob and me. Hadn't she been listening? Had she missed the fact that he'd been ready to put her horse down before I presented another option? To top it off, we never even got paid for the pharmaceuticals I had given him. I guess Miss Marshall and Doc Bob both felt I was fortunate just to have been in his presence.

A Cat on the Counter

Fred had a reputation that preceded her. Yes, her. She had originally been brought into the clinic, long before I came along, for a routine male neutering procedure. It quickly became obvious that the parts that were meant to be removed were not there. This confusion is common when it comes to young kittens, since it can be hard for owners to distinguish gender. Then, once the sex is decided on and a name is given, there is no reason to question. At any rate, the surgical instruments were quickly exchanged for those required for a cat spay, and Fred became a neutered female.

The long-term problem was that over the years Fred had grown to hate her trips to the clinic. I don't know if it started with the original mix-up or just built up over time, but she really despised it and was now beginning to take this attitude out on her owners and the staff. It had gotten to the point that, when we saw Fred's name on the schedule, we would consider faking a sick day just to avoid the risk of personal injury.

Then one day, Fred's owner, Mrs. Umbaugh, called me to talk about the situation with Fred. "I was wondering if because of Fred's aversion to going to the clinic, it would be possible for you to come to our house to see Fred," she said. I paused, then replied carefully, "That might not be a bad idea. Let's make an appointment and I will stop by and give it a try." All she needed was some vaccinations, but in the case of Fred, even the most routine procedure could turn into a big ordeal.

The appointment was set up for the following Friday morning, so Jenny and I headed over to the Umbaughs'. We really didn't know what to expect from Fred on her home turf, so we armed ourselves with thick leather gloves and heavy jackets. We pulled in the narrow driveway, where snow was piled along the sides from the last storm. Gathering the necessary syringes, vaccine, and personal armor, we tromped through snow to the front door of the spacious home. Mrs. Umbaugh came to the tall oak door with curlers in her dark hair and her robe still on. She was a small woman with a warm smile and big brown eyes. Her husband was an airline pilot and they had met when she was working as a flight attendant. Mr. Umbaugh was gone a lot due to his work, so she and Fred were pretty close. "Oh, thank you so much for coming!" she exclaimed. "I just know that she will be happier here." We headed into the living room, where Fred was patiently waiting on the couch. The last thing in the world she expected was to see us on her home turf. The shock lasted just long enough for Mrs. Umbaugh to grab her, keeping the feline from disappearing under the furniture. We decided that the kitchen counter would be the best substitute for an exam table, so Mrs. Umbaugh headed into the voluminous kitchen, with Jenny and me in tow. She placed Fred on the granite countertop and turned her over to Jenny. I examined Fred and listened to her heart and lungs with my stethoscope. Then I pulled up the vaccine and headed toward Fred with a syringe. This was when she decided that needles were evil whether at home or in the clinic. She emitted a low growl, the kind that should have come only from a full-grown lion, not a ten-pound kitty on a kitchen counter.

At this point, we seemed to be in no better situation than if we had been in the clinic. Then Jenny came up with an idea. "When I was in veterinary technician school, one of my teachers showed me a little trick that might just work on Fred." She smiled wisely as she continued to explain. "If I push Fred along the counter from behind, she might concentrate on where she is going more than on what you are doing to her." The counter in the Umbaughs' kitchen was very long and made a ninety-degree turn near the end, giving it an L shape. We all agreed that this technique would be worth a try, so we prepared to put the plan into action.

We moved Fred to the end of the countertop, the farthest end from the sharp turn. I was ready with loaded syringes and Jenny stood beside the counter with her hands positioned on each side of Fred's haunches. We knew that the procedure would have to be performed quickly, because even though the counter was long, there was only so much of it. Jenny began pushing her along and I started vaccinating. Mrs. Umbaugh kept her fingers crossed. Sure enough, it appeared to be working. Fred plunked down her rear end and put her front legs out in front of her. She was trying to stop the forward motion with her spread front paws and was concentrating so hard that she didn't notice the needles. I had completed two injections by the time Fred had reached the turn on the counter, and I had one left to go. Jenny maneuvered Fred around the tight corner, giving me just enough time to finish the job. Suddenly, it was all over. No mortal flesh wounds, no upset kitty, and, most fortunately, no excrement. Mrs. Umbaugh just stared in amazement. "I can't believe it. This is the greatest!" she yelled as she gave her cat a big hug. But the most amazed was Fred. She sat there in total astonishment, receiving love from her owner. Her expression indicated she was almost disappointed that she had just been through a full set of cat vaccinations and not even had a chance to object.

Jenny beamed with pride at the success of her suggestion, and I knew I would be buying her lunch to reward her for her ingenuity. I didn't mind at all, since I had been dreading this house call from the day we had made the arrangements. We victoriously packed up our things and headed back for the truck. Mrs. Umbaugh thanked us profusely, waving from the doorway as we drove up the driveway to the main road. Jenny and I heaved big sighs of relief once we were out of sight, and I bought lunch at the restaurant of her choice.

We returned to the Umbaughs' three or four times over the next couple of years for minor injuries and vaccinations. We even had to open an abscess on the countertop once. I never ate any of the baked goods Mrs. Umbaugh offered me after that. Fred seemed to be leading the life of a normal, healthy cat, but then one day Mrs. Umbaugh called in and said she was very concerned. Fred had not been acting like herself lately and her appetite was decreasing daily. I went over and examined Fred on the counter, listening to her heart, lungs, and palpating for lumps and bumps. Fred was too cooperative, hardly putting up a fuss at all. I was conversing with Mrs. Umbaugh about everyday things like the weather when I came across a lump in the area of Fred's mammary glands. Jenny rolled Fred on her side and, sure enough, I found not just one mass but two. I suspected Fred had mammary cancer (similar to breast cancer in humans), a very aggressive cancer in cats. "What is it?" Mrs. Umbaugh asked. The fact that that I had stopped participating in the conversation so abruptly clued her in that I had found something. "We have found a couple masses here on the belly area," I said, trying to draw Jenny into sharing the blame. "Do you mean cancerous tumors?" she asked cautiously. I paused a second, but there was no way to sugarcoat the answer. "Most probably," I finally managed to say. "We will need to do some X rays to see if it has spread to any other areas." Mrs. Umbaugh's eyes were beginning to moisten now and she just shook her head to give us the go-ahead.

Normally, we would have to x-ray cats in the clinic, but this situation was becoming more sensitive by the minute. Taking Fred to the clinic at this point would just have put more stress on her and Mrs. Umbaugh. Jenny and I showed up two days later with the large-animal portable X-ray machine. We put Fred through the usual counter routine in order to sedate her for the X rays. We set up the whole apparatus outside, donned our lead protective gear, and calibrated the machine for a small cat. We took the sleepy Fred outdoors to our temporary radiology department. Then after taking the appropriate shots of her chest and abdomen, we returned her to her luxury purple cat bed in the corner of the living room to sleep it off. "We'll have the results for you later this afternoon. We will call you and you can meet us at the clinic to look at the X rays," I told Mrs. Umbaugh, secretly dreading what we might find.

We loaded up our equipment and headed back to the clinic. While I saw some more clients over the noon hour, Jenny developed the X rays. When they were done, she put them up on the X-ray viewer in the treatment room, checking them over herself before I had a chance to look. As I walked into the room, Jenny shook her head sadly. "Doesn't look good." She grimaced. I could see the problems well before I reached the viewer. The lungs were covered with little white spots, each the size of a pencil eraser, and the liver had a few of the same lesions developing. The cancer had already spread to other organs.

Before we called Mrs. Umbaugh, I phoned a veterinary oncologist at the veterinary college to see if she had any ideas. She ran through a short list of chemotherapy agents that could be used for cancer in cats. She then cautioned that none would work well in cats with cancer this severe and might cause the animal undue discomfort, with little benefit.

Jenny called Mrs. Umbaugh to ask her to come in and I tried to prepare myself to give her the bad news. When she arrived, Jenny led her over to the viewer and I proceeded to show her what was going on. The tears flowed down her face, taking her makeup with them as I told her what the oncologist had relayed to me. She stared at Fred's X rays for a few minutes before managing to say, "Fred would not do well with regular treatments. Is there anything we could give her to keep her comfortable for now?" I had Jenny put together some cortisone tablets to make Fred's life a little easier. Then, just before Mrs. Umbaugh walked out the door, she looked at me and attempted to speak. I spoke first so that she didn't have to ask. "You will know when it is time. She will let you know." Mrs. Umbaugh nodded her head knowingly and headed home to spend time with Fred.

Mrs. Umbaugh let us know a few days later that Fred had picked up just a bit, but we all knew that this was a temporary effect from the cortisone drugs. Jenny and I went on with our usual workdays and put Fred in the back of our minds for a little while. Mrs. Umbaugh called about three weeks after we had done the X rays. The shaky voice on the other end of the line said, "You said I would know when, and it's now." Jenny and I headed over to the Umbaughs' that afternoon. This is always the worst part of the job, but we knew it needed to be done for Fred's sake. Inside the house, I explained that we would first give Fred a sedative to make the whole process easier on her. Then, after she was relaxed, I would administer the euthanasia solution into the vein in her front leg. Even a debilitated Fred would fight the intravenous injection if we didn't sedate her first.

I was just ready to get started, when I realized that Mr. Umbaugh was not present and that Mrs. Umbaugh could really use him right now. I knew he was gone a lot, but I thought that today he would have tried to be home. "Is Mr. Umbaugh around today?" I asked. A worse question could not have been asked. She immediately broke into uncontrollable crying. Mr. Umbaugh had recently left her for a younger flight attendant. Jenny gave me a disgusted look, as if I should have known better. I didn't know what else to do but give Mrs. Umbaugh a hug and hold her until she could gather herself. She then gave me a nod and we continued with our task.

Jenny and Fred began their last trip down the long counter. I slipped the sedative into Fred and in a few minutes she was sleeping quietly. Mrs. Umbaugh stroked her fur as I injected the euthanasia solution. In a matter of seconds, Fred was gone and out of her discomfort. Mrs. Umbaugh said her final good-bye and kissed Fred on the top of the head. We wrapped her in her favorite blanket and placed her in her cat bed. A neighbor was coming over later to help her bury Fred in the backyard. She gave us each a final hug on the way out and thanked us for all of our past help in making Fred's life easier.

Back in the truck, Jenny and I didn't even look at each other. Eventually, she broke the silence. "I'd like to kick Mr. Umbaugh hard," she muttered. I agreed and we continued down the road, making innocuous conversation to take our minds off the situation. It seemed that Mrs. Umbaugh had just been overwhelmed with bad fortune and we had been a part of it.

A few days later, I received a note in the mail thanking Jenny and me for all of our help at a difficult time. Mrs. Umbaugh also thanked us for all the times we had made a special effort to come out and treat Fred on the countertop. The letter made me feel a little better. We had just done what was necessary and what was best for Fred, but it had obviously meant a lot to Mrs. Umbaugh.

Often people who lose a pet don't want to start looking for a new one right away. They will often say, "It is just too hard. I can't stand the thought of getting attached and losing another pet." Some people need more time for grieving than others do. Inevitably, another pet will find its way into a person's life when the timing is right.

In the case of Mrs. Umbaugh, that time came about six months later, when she was shopping at the local grocery store. Such stores are often a social center in a lot of Dakota communities. That day, a family with a cardboard box full of squirmy brown-and-white puppies was hoping to find them good homes. The puppies were the product of a synchronized escape by a male Border collie and a female Welsh corgi from their respective backyards. The owners of the corgi were the ones left holding the vegetable box, now responsible for finding new homes for the pups. Mrs. Umbaugh tried not to look at the box of fuzz balls as she picked up her pace. Knowing her own weakness, she dreaded having to leave the store, and she attempted to turn her head to avoid the squeaking little urchins. But by this time, they had spilled out of the box and were crawling around in front of the store. There they were, right in front of her, making it hard just to run by. In fact, she nearly stepped on a particularly small one. He looked up at her pitifully and wagged his stubby little tail, using his God-given equipment and talent to draw in a human. Mrs. Umbaugh bent over to pick him up and never let go.

When she brought Fredrick in for his first puppy shots, I was surprised to see her with a new pet, let alone a canine. Yet the biggest surprise was that she also had a new man. He had not rolled out of a cardboard box in front of a storefront. They had met at a benefit for a humane organization and their mutual love for animals brought them together. He appeared to be a very nice fellow and seemed to care very much for Mrs. Umbaugh. Even so, I never wanted anything to do with him as a client. Snakes were his pets of choice.

Do No Harm

One of the toughest ways to make a living, in my opinion, is dairy farming. Although a number of dairies are corporate-owned and -managed these days, many family-owned facilities remain across the United States. These struggling farmers are constantly dealing with the rise and fall of milk prices, feed costs, and disease. Eastern South Dakota still has a fairly large concentration of these hardworking folks and their cows.

From a veterinarian's standpoint, working on dairy cows can be both rewarding and exhausting at the same time. Most farmers milk their cows three times a day. This schedule keeps the cows the most comfortable while also allowing the maximum amount of milk to be retrieved from each one. The only problem with this schedule is that to get in three milkings, the farmers have to get started really early and finish the last one at around seven to eight o'clock at night. I found out early on that after this last milking was when a farmer would call me if he had a problem—around 8:00 P.M., when he went into the house. So by the time I got out of my television-watching clothes and into something appropriate for a dairy barn, I might be able to get there by 9:00 P.M. Depending on how far away they were, it might be even later.

I also began to realize that besides being there to treat a problem, I was often the evening entertainment. After a night of *Young Veterinarian on Trial,* they could catch the ten o'clock news and go to bed satisfied. Summer was not the best time to be in a midwestern dairy barn. They were usually kept very clean and tidy, but it took only a little bit of spilled milk to make the whole place smell sour in the humid prairie heat.

On one particular July evening, Jenny and I were more than ready to go home, having worked hard all day. Since the air conditioning in the truck was on the fritz, sweat had soaked through our clothes hours before. We were about a mile away from the clinic when the two-way radio crackled. "Mr. Abel has a cow down. He wants you there right away. He insists that this cow be seen tonight, or he will call someone else."

Mr. Abel and his wife were in their late sixties but in great shape. They were strong and showed hardly any signs of age-related diseases. Their good health could probably be attributed to a life of hard work and an endless supply of milk. Tom Abel was also known as the tightest man in the county, so needless to say, we didn't see the Abels very often. The only times we did were when an animal was near death.

The red summer sun was just starting to go down behind the silos when we pulled into the run-down barnyard. The minute I opened the door of my truck, we could hear the patient's breathing above all the other farm noise and knew we were in trouble. The old cow was tied to the side of the barn, with her front legs spread to allow for maximum air intake. I started to examine her, when Tom came storming through the corral, wife in tow. "I don't want to spend a lot of money; she's my lowest producer. I don't know why I'm even messing with her," he said in his most condescending tone.

I raised my eyes from my stethoscope just enough to acknowledge his presence, then continued to listen to her lungs. I could tell she had something blocking her windpipe, possibly a tumor or abscess. On examining her mouth, I realized she might have been the oldest living cow on record and had fewer teeth than Mr. Abel. Finally, I stated the obvious, announcing, "She doesn't look too good." Tom responded proudly, "The last veterinarian treated her for the same problem and she was much better by morning."

I wanted to say, Well, why didn't you call that vet again? but I refrained. Eventually, I came up with a plan to try to at least temporarily relieve her breathing problem.

After I explained to Mr. Able that we needed to give the old girl some IV antibiotics and antiinflammatory drugs, he squinted his eyes, staring at me with detectable doubt. "She's a wild one," he said. "I don't know how you'll manage to restrain her."

I suggested that we take her into the milking parlor, where we could put her in a stall to keep her relatively still. But Tom informed us that she would tear up the parlor if we attempted to do this. I was running out of ideas when I happened to think that we could just lay her down with an arrangement of ropes and keep her that way long enough to give her the IV medication. Tom gave an approving nod to this procedure, and Jenny grabbed the cotton rope from the truck.

Using the rope, we easily got her down and began the last-ditch treatment to try to save her. I was relieved to see fresh red blood bubble out of the catheter when I slid it under the skin in the general direction of the jugular vein. Attaching a bottle of medication to the catheter with plastic tubing, I held the bottle above her, allowing it to run in at the appropriate pace. After a couple of minutes of conversation to pass the time while the treatment continued, Jenny jabbed me in the ribs with her elbow and pointed at the cow. She called my attention to a situation that I had just begun to notice. The patient had not recently moved or taken a breath. I pressed my stethoscope against the chest wall and could find no heartbeat. Her gums were purple and her pupils dilated. The stress of the treatment had been just enough to put her over the edge.

Mr. Abel had been spewing his opinion on the politics of the day, not noticing the stricken look on our faces. "Tom," I said, interrupting him, "we've lost her." He stopped in the middle of a dissertation on Reaganomics and stared blankly at the dead cow. I explained that she had just been in too bad shape to survive and that I was very sorry.

All four of us stood staring at the lifeless animal for an uncomfortably long time. Finally, Tom shook his head and acknowledged that she probably would not have recovered anyway, given that she had died this easily. As we put our equipment back into the truck, I felt that all had ended as well as it could have, considering that the patient hadn't made it. At least she was out of her misery. We headed back to the clinic, stopping at the Dairy Queen for chocolate shakes to drown our sorrows.

The next morning, I stopped at the local Casey's for gas a little before 8:00 A.M. and noticed Johnny, the owner, rushing out the door to greet me. He had a suspiciously large grin on his face, as he often did when he had some juicy local gossip. That day, it was about me. "Hey, Doc, I hear that you killed Tom Abel's best cow," Johnny yelled across the pumps. "He said that she was fine until you got to her."

Tom had already been in that morning and told him this rather imaginative version of the story. "Yeah, told me he didn't know how he would be able to stay in business without the milk produced by that invaluable cow."

I tried to melt into the pavement, but there was no escape. Johnny had a big old belly laugh over my distress before finally leaning over to whisper in my ear. "Don't worry," he said, "no one has believed anything Tom has said in over thirty years."

Rocky Mountain High

At the end of my second year of practice, I decided that I could not spend another winter in the Dakotas, and I heard the call of the Rocky Mountains. Having spent several summers in Colorado, I missed the mountains and the outdoor lifestyle that goes with them.

One of those summers, I had worked with a veterinarian in a mixed-animal practice to get some hands-on experience. We had talked on the phone several times that spring, while I was still in South Dakota, and he had eventually offered me a job. It was hard to say good-bye to Jenny and the rest of the staff, but the thought of the upcoming prairie winds and horizontal snowstorms made it a little easier. Winter in the upper Midwest creates a lifestyle that has many similarities to the hibernation of bears. People tend to stay in their houses and peek through their iced-up windows, wondering if the sun has forsaken them for eternity. For some reason, those who have grown up in the Dakotas don't seem to care. They don't mind scraping a full inch of solid ice off their car windshields every morning, or the fact that all vehicles have electrical cords hanging from their engine blocks so they'll start the next day. The leathery, creased faces of the farmers are testament to what they endure.

With all this in mind, I loaded up a plywood-sided, open-topped trailer, hitched it to my 1977 Jeep Cherokee (the one that actually had the metallic Indian chief on the side), and headed southwest for Colorado. At twenty-eight I had very little to hold me down—no serious relationships or home ownership, but no money, either. This made it extra painful when my vacuum cleaner and microwave blew out of my trailer and exploded on the pavement somewhere in eastern Nebraska. Considering that I still had high student-loan payments and was only earning a beginning veterinarian's salary, these items would not be replaced soon. I had not put away any money during the previous year and a half, so by the time I reached the snowcapped peaks, I was completely broke. I had just enough to make an apartment deposit and pay the first month's rent, but that was it. I wouldn't get my first paycheck for two weeks, and I had only twenty dollars to my name. This time was a little stressful, until I discovered the Little Debbie cookies sandwich. For those who don't know, it consists of two oatmeal cookies with a kind of whipped cream in the middle. I could buy a box of one dozen for a dollar, and preparation was minimal—just open the bag. On special nights, I would splurge with a side of ramen noodles, an extra ten cents.

My tiny cabin was very basic but came with a great view of Pikes Peak. The cabin consisted of a main floor with a rustic living room, bathroom, and kitchen. At one end of the main floor, a homemade wooden ladder led up to a sleeping loft. I learned quickly that I needed to give myself plenty of time to make it down to the bathroom in the middle of the night. Excessive caffeine late in the day made for some frantic rappelling in the dark. These were tight quarters, but the beautiful views and ever-present deer in the driveway made it a great place to come home to.

I furnished the cabin with vintage lawn chairs from a local yard sale, the best I could do on my young practitioner's budget. As you can imagine, this type of interior decorating really impressed the young ladies. Bad taste aside, with the twelve-dollar wooden-framed console television, purchased during college, it made a reasonable bachelor pad, although I did miss my vacuum and microwave. It would have been nice to warm up my Little Debbie sandwiches occasionally. When that first modest paycheck came around, I felt like a Rockefeller and headed directly for the food market.

Unlike the elaborate veterinary clinics in larger cities, rural mountain clinics tend to be rather inconspicuous, and this one was no exception. It was a small one-story wood-sided building that had obviously been added onto more than once. The carpet in the waiting room had been around a little too long, absorbing the odors of excrement that nervous patients had left behind. A little examination room had doors leading to an X-ray area, laboratory, and a treatment/surgery room with stainless-steel kennels, where patients could sleep off anesthesia. The doctors' office was tucked in the back and equipped with a door to the outside in case a quick escape was warranted. Outdoors, the scent of huge old ponderosa pines provided relief from any stressful events that might have occurred during the workday.

The gravel driveway ran directly from the highway about one-half the length of a city block to a four-car parking lot beside the front door. It had just enough of an uphill grade to require four-wheel drive on a snowy day. Those clients without it would have to leave their vehicles at the bottom and hike to the top. When the snow began to melt, the driveway became more of a luge course than a driveway, and it often shot clients back onto the highway a little faster than they had planned. But for all of its shortcomings, the clinic contained all that we needed to do a good job of caring for our patients and their owners.

Changing jobs not only means new surroundings; it also requires getting to know a new staff. In the veterinary profession, these people are not just fellow workers; they become practically family after you have spent uncountable twelve-hour days together. All and all, they had better be people you can get along with, or those long hours will seem like years.

When I walked into work the first day, Lorraine, the receptionist, gazed at me from behind the narrow countertop that was her personal domain. At first, she looked a little puzzled, then realized who I was and perked up. "Well, glad to see you could make it" were her first words. I guess I was a few minutes late. "Christie needs some help in the back." A bony finger pointed the way, and I obeyed unquestioningly. Lorraine was in her early fifties. She had sunken eyes and long dark hair with frequent streaks of gray—obviously, she had given up on dying it many years before. She now wore her gray locks like a badge of honor that gave her the right to dole out orders to all of us. She was the first line of defense at the clinic. Everyone and every situation had to get past her before we became involved.

In the treatment room, I found my new technician/assistant covered with putrid brown diarrhea. A young Chesapeake retriever had gotten into his owners' kitchen garbage while they were sleeping. As luck would have it, the garbage had contained a pot of leftover chili that had been abandoned in the fridge long enough to grow its own shell of greenish mold. Much to the humans' disappointment, they had discovered their pup's illness while making breakfast barefoot in the kitchen that morning. The children had needed a second shower before leaving for school.

Christie had made the mistake of picking up the nauseated dog to transfer it to the treatment area and had put a little too much pressure on the animal's abdomen. Projectile diarrhea on clean clothes would make most people more than a little upset, but she was obviously a dedicated caregiver and appeared to be unshaken by her soiled clothing or splattered face.

Christie was only twenty years old, but that day she looked much older than her years. Dog feces don't tend to give people a youthful appearance. She was blond, slight of build, and was rather attractive most days. Finding myself at a loss for words that morning, I mumbled, "Anything I can do to help?" Eventually, she broke into a sheepish smile and wiped her hand off on her pants before jamming it out to shake mine. I hesitated, but realizing this was a test to see how squeamish the new guy was, I grabbed it and shook it vigorously. "Nice to finally meet you. Can I get the name of that perfume?" I asked.

She snickered a little and replied, "Oh, don't worry, I'm sure you'll be wearing some of your own soon enough." Then she turned on her heel and headed to the rest room to clean up. I took that chance to use the sink in the treatment room to wash my hands. Dog feces in the morning still makes me gag a little, especially on an empty stomach.

We would later laugh repeatedly about that first meeting. There would be many days ahead when we both would find ourselves covered in horse manure, cow placenta, or dog vomit. These are just hazards of the job, which when endured together make for some great friendships.

City Slickers

Once in a while in veterinary practice, you get to do something out of the ordinary and adventuresome. One beautiful Rocky Mountain fall day happened to be one of those times. A rancher client had called in right after the office opened, upset that one of the neighbor's male buffalo had gotten in with his cattle. Apparently, the bison's bravado was keeping the big boy from returning home. A group of wanna-be cowboys had attempted a roundup, but they found the bull to be a bit more determined than their suburban mounts. Fortunately, the rancher explained, no one had died yet.

My client's fear lay, of course, in the next year's crop of calves. Left too long with his cows, the buffalo would see to a new herd of "beefalo" being delivered next spring. These would not be as valuable at auction as his purebred cattle and could cause a true financial crisis for my client.

Now, where do I come in? you ask. Have you ever seen Mutual of Omaha's *Wild Kingdom?* My client requested I come quick and dart this errant buffalo with a tranquilizer so the owner could get him into a trailer. This was living! I loaded up the tranquilizer gun and eagerly hopped in the truck to head to the ranch.

A vast landscape of high alpine pastures and groups of evergreens opened up before me. The ranch had been in this family for generations, tucked away in a remote region served by the practice. I shook myself free of the visions of playing Jim, the Marlin Perkins sidekick, with my body half out of a speeding Land Rover, aiming at an angry Cape buffalo.

The large sign as I turned off the dusty road read KUGLER PURE-BRED HEREFORD RANCH. Another sign with a *K* set on rockers, revealing the family's Rocking K Ranch brand, hung at the ranch entrance. A cattle guard shook the truck cab as I pulled up to the house. The dust cloud I created temporarily obscured a motley-looking crew of greenhorn ranch hands, who appeared to be discouraged.

I had barely unfolded myself from the truck when I was met by the owner of the buffalo. Mr. Seldon was a tall, disheveled man with deep-set eyes. I didn't know him personally but had heard he'd transplanted himself here from New York twenty years earlier with the dream of raising buffalo. He briefly glanced my way and then grunted, "I don't want you to hurt him—just slow him down a bit." Over his shoulder a two-thousand-pound bull bison appeared in the distance. From my vantage point, he looked like an army tank with horns, and my last concern was my hurting him.

The plan conceived before my arrival was to drive the big boy past a broken-down shed that I would be hiding in. At the precise moment, I would take aim and hit him with the dart. Precision was the key. I had to load the dart with just the right dosage of drug. Too little would just make him mad, and too much might kill him. If I missed—well, that just wasn't an option.

I watched the "cowboys" begin to gather, sporting their lassos and appearing intent on using them. I warned them that if they agitated the bull by throwing the ropes too soon, the sedation would have a reverse effect. They nodded in slow agreement. I preferred that they simply walk behind him after the sedation took effect and gently coax him toward the trailer. They did not nod their heads in agreement with this. What kind of a macho war story ended with "and as we coaxed him to the trailer . . ."? No! They imagined dragging the beast behind them in victory. I couldn't allow them to get hurt. I imagined my vet school classmates shaking their heads in shock and disapproval as they read about it in the monthly liability reports in the veterinary journals.

It was time to commence the plan. I knelt in the shed and waited for the cattle to amble by. I have to admit that I may briefly have imagined myself in a fringed buckskin jacket, ready to fell a buffalo to bring back to the hungry pioneers. Back to reality, though, there he was, just twenty feet away, slowly following the cows. I second-guessed my sedation dose. Was it too much? Not enough? It was too late now. I peered through the crosshairs and pulled the trigger as he came into view. I heard the low thump of the dart hitting the tough hide and saw his agitated kick. A direct hit! I almost went into a touchdown dance but then decided to act as if I had expected no other outcome.

Everything was going according to plan. Our shaggy friend began to slow and get wobbly, as if he'd had one too many martinis. Within a minute, the great beast lay down, and I began to pack up and head to the truck. My work here was done. Quick, precise, and clean. The whole episode had gone off like a perfectly executed fourth-down play.

Suddenly, a roar went up from the cowboy crowd. Yes, one of them had thrown a rope on the bull, yanking him back into reality.

Throwing the rope around the fading animal's neck caused him to spring up and tear off into the woods with the rope dragging behind.

I felt I couldn't leave until the animal was again subdued. I grabbed a second lasso out of the truck and headed for the woods with no particular plan—just complete agitation with the now-sheepish-looking group of "helpers." The bull was up and running but still a little sedated. The idea came to me that I could tie my rope to the one he was already wearing and possibly recapture him. Running through the pine trees after him, I must have looked like an idiot. But he eventually slowed just enough for me to grab the end of his rope. Using some Boy Scout ingenuity, I lashed the two ends of rope together in a square knot while keeping pace with the fleeing beast. This left a long-enough expanse to tie him off to a tree, but I was not taking into consideration what he would do when he hit the end of his new leash.

In a split second, he hit the end of the rope, and it stretched like a bungee cord. The tree groaned under the tension, but the hundred-year-old roots held fast. At this point, my worst fears were realized. He began to turn toward me and lower his head. I was almost too tired to care, until he began to charge. I sprinted away from him, grabbed my tranquilizer gun, and headed for the truck. He was right on my heals when he ran out of rope for the second time. Now my work here was truly done. Speeding away, I waved and yelled a hearty "Good luck!" out the window.

Over the next couple of weeks, I wondered what had happened to the buffalo and his handlers after I left the ranch. Then one morning as I was heading toward the bank, Mr. Seldon came out of the building. He was walking with a limp, which I didn't remember him having before, and his left hand was wrapped in a bandage. He waved when he saw me. "Hey, Doc, thanks for all your help with that bison. We got him home safe and sound." Then he slid into his old truck and took off. I didn't have the heart to ask how he'd gotten the injuries, but since we hadn't received any calls from attorneys, I felt it best not to know.

Seemed Like a Good Idea

 Animals so often display traits that I truly admire. Ignoring the force of terrifying foes, they press on, denying their battle-weary bodies rest until the job is done. Animals can be extremely tenacious, especially when it comes to taking on other beasts. For some reason, porcupines seem to bring out this "never give in" attitude in their opponents more than any other species.

How many times have I witnessed the results of canine-versus-porcupine encounters and ended up treating them? Cats rarely end up in this predicament, since they are usually smart enough not to make such a painful mistake.

Contrary to popular opinion, porcupines don't "shoot" quills at everything that moves. In fact, in order for a quill to find itself in another being, the potential predator has to make contact with the porcupine. These spike-covered creatures move very slowly, like a drunk who takes every step with concentration and deliberation.

They are not really capable of running, so when attacked, they just curl up in a ball, as if to dare predators to take a bite. Any animal naïve enough to try to eat them will end up with a face full of quills. Man's best friend seems to be the most common animal to fall into this category.

The most pitiful porcupine victim I have ever treated had five hundred quills carpeting the roof of its mouth, as well as its nose and paws. After a couple hours of surgery, the dog was quill-free, but he visited me eleven more times for repeat offenses over the next few years. It is just a myth that dogs learn from such a miserable experience.

My most memorable victims of a porcupine's wrath were three Jack Russell terriers who hailed from a remote mountain area called "the park," about an hour from the clinic. The Jack Russell is the definition of a big dog in a little-dog suit. They all behave as if someone forgot to tell them they are small. On a summer Sunday afternoon about one o'clock, Mrs. Conner, the owner of these three Jack Russells, called in a panic because the entire crew had attacked a porcupine. She was leaving immediately, bound for the clinic.

Mrs. Conner was a small but determined woman of about forty-five. She seemed a perfect match for the canine breed she had selected as pets. When they arrived, the three musketeers were pretty proud of themselves. Each one had about twenty well-placed spikes in the end of its nose and came prancing in as if the quills were trophies.

"I can't believe all three got so many quills!" Mrs. Conner exclaimed. Then, to her dogs, she added, "There are easier ways to attract attention to yourself, you know!"

One by one, they lined up proudly, practically refusing sedation. Each one stood like a statue on the exam table, too macho to show pain, until it finally sat, sedated. Mrs. Conner held them and soothed them while I worked. Her slight hands made the magisterial terriers look, and probably feel, much bigger than they really were.

Slowly, every quill was removed from the now-sleepy terriers with a quick tug. The dogs were given back to their owner, no worse for wear. Within minutes, they were harassing the clinic cats. I sent them home with sore noses and antibiotics. I finally returned to my basement apartment to finish my Hungry Man meal and catch a Sunday afternoon nap.

A little after four o'clock, my pager went off, and I sleepily fumbled for the phone. It was Mrs. Conner again, but this time there was frustration, not fear, in her voice. Through clenched teeth, she said, seething, "They finished him off this time, and I'm on the way back in!" Slam went the phone in my ear. An hour later, I gave her wide berth as she flew through the familiar clinic doorway. Under both arms were tucked the exuberant terriers, faces completely full of the silvery spikes this time. Evidently, these dogs had taken out a little vengeance on their porcupine friend, and they were again proud of the results.

General anesthesia was required for removing this many quills, so it was a couple of hours before they were once again released to their exasperated owner. Mrs. Conner glared at the bill, then turned to her groggy little friends. "So how do you plan to pay for this?" she asked them sternly. They responded with only somnolent smiles and wagging tongues, eagerly awaiting their next adventure even in their dreams. I heard later that the terriers spent the next two weeks "grounded" in the garage.

Occupational Hazard

Veterinary practice can be a dangerous endeavor. There is always the risk of dog and cat bites, which may be induced either by fear or by the pain that your treatment might cause them. Although these wounds are sometimes very painful and may produce a lot of veterinarian blood, they are not often life-threatening. It is the large-animal side of practice that can require an increase in life insurance. I have been chased by a multitude of cows, spitting llamas, and even an occasional upset sheep, but the horse has probably been the animal to come closest to ending my career.

I have always had a great fondness for horses, and we were lucky enough to have them as pets when I was growing up, starting with dear old Midge, the wonderful Welsh pony. These early experiences allowed me to develop a huge amount of respect for these beautiful, powerful creatures. It is amazing to reflect on the role horses played in developing civilization up until just a hundred years ago. We humans could never have done it without them, but most of them are now relegated to the position of pets and or recreational animals. Unfortunately, since we live in a society that no longer requires the daily use of horses, not only are horse owners able to spend less time with their steeds but some owners are not well equipped to deal with these animals. Most of my clients do a great job of training and caring for their equine companions, making my dealings with them an enjoyable experience, but every so often a horse comes along that is less than pleased to see me.

A prime example of unruly patients occurred on a brisk Colorado spring day when I headed out to see a new horse client. Calling on familiar clients, you know what you're getting into with both the horses and the humans, but this was not the case that day. As I stopped the truck in front of the typical cedar-sided mountain home, a small-framed, smiling woman of about thirty-five with long dark hair and cowboy boots came up from the barn. She stuck out her hand and introduced herself as Jane Scott, a newcomer in the community. She appeared to be genuinely happy to meet another resident of the county and introduced the two grade school–age children peering shyly at me from behind her. After a lame attempt at making friends with the youngsters, I loaded up with vaccine and followed the group toward the stable. They had five horses, four in neat, clean stalls and an especially large one pacing nervously in a high-fenced round pen outside. Jane suggested that we take care of the stalled horses first, so I took her advice and we headed into the barn. The patients were four beautiful, well-mannered quarter horses, all of whom stood perfectly still while I examined and vaccinated them. I noticed that Jane was becoming a little nervous as we finished up with the last shiny, freshly groomed animal. I gathered up my supplies and we headed back outside to complete the task.

The children, who had seemed to enjoy observing the shots their pets had to endure in the barn, now made a break for the house, disappearing through the back door. About this time, I noticed that the buckskin horse we were approaching was not diligently well groomed like the other horses. In fact, he was rather shaggy and unkempt. As we approached, Jane's pace slowed, and when she stopped in front of the pen, we both stared at the big horse in front of us. She looked down at her feet, kicking the dust as she spoke. "I always meant to have him gelded but never really got around to it," she said. She went on to tell me that Rebel was now nine years old and hadn't been worked with much. Jane indicated that they just hadn't had the time to spend with him, but I was beginning to surmise that he might not be that easy to be around. A nine-year-old untrained stallion was going to be a formidable patient.

Jane was trying to hide her tremors as I followed her into the corral. "I really need to get him vaccinated; it's been a couple years," she said sheepishly. Then she added reluctantly, "The last vet wouldn't come back." Her dark eyes glanced in my direction to look for a reaction.

I knew that I could not show fear, because both she and the horse were looking for any sign of weakness. The big guy snorted and shook his head as we entered his domain. I swallowed hard when the heavy metal gate slammed shut behind me; now we were committed, or so I thought. Jane stood on tiptoes. She clipped the lead rope onto the halter and handed it to me so Rebel and I could get acquainted before I attempted any vaccinations. Talking softy, I attempted to move in closer to gain his trust. "Easy, big guy, let's take it easy," I whispered while trying not to falter.

He stared me down for a moment, then blew out all the air from his lungs through his nasal passages, producing a startling snort and nearly knocking off my hat. Jane's anxiety seemed to increase even more, and she kept looking around as if hoping to locate an escape route. It was officially a standoff. The next move was mine, so I reached into my pocket and drew out my stethoscope. With the earpieces in place, I moved in to listen to his heart, but Rebel took this as an act of aggression and reared up on his back legs, striking out at us with his front hooves. I dodged to the side just in time to see Jane slide under the fence and sprint for the deck at the rear of the house. Upon reaching her destination, she turned and yelled back, gasping for breath at the same time, "I think he'll be better without me in there."

Now it was just me and the thirteen-hundred-pound testosterone-filled equine. I decided to assume that his heart and lungs were fine and go right for the shots. He seemed to be all muscle and hooves as he bucked and charged around the pen after recognizing the syringes I pulled out of my pocket. I managed to keep hold of the lead rope, even though he would charge me, teeth bared, every thirty seconds. What I really wanted to do was follow Jane's lead and make a mad dash for the safety of the house. But I had to stay and get the job done. I couldn't show weakness, especially in front of a new client. It was one of those moments when I felt as if the rest of the world had fallen away and all that existed was the horse and me.

Trying to accept that I would most likely be killed by this upset animal, I just let him continue circling around me. Much to my surprise, he eventually began to slow down. The big horse was beginning to wear out. Finally, the stallion came to a stop and turned to face me, but this time he didn't attempt to charge; he just stood quietly, covered with sweat. His eyes were focused directly on me, yet the anger was gone and a soft look of submission had replaced it. I moved toward him cautiously, waiting for an explosion of teeth and hooves. Again I was surprised that it didn't happen, even when I produced the syringes again. Rebel let me rub him on the side of his neck with the palm of my hand and assure him quietly as the needles found their target in the large muscles of his neck. At last he was vaccinated, and he even let me check his teeth, heart, and lungs without objection.

Jane had her hand covering her eyes while she peeked between her fingers, as if she were watching a scene in a scary movie that she didn't want to look at but couldn't resist. I'm sure she didn't think I would live through it. After taking off the halter, I went over and handed it to her and we settled up. She seemed happy to pay the bill, since Rebel had actually gotten his vaccines this time, and I was just glad to have survived. In fact, I had a little fantasy about seeing a moving van in front of their house before vaccination time the following spring.

As lucky as I was not to have been damaged this time, my next encounter with an upset equine would not have such a happy ending.

The next few weeks of spring vaccinations went by without incident. All the horses were cooperative and well mannered, but a call came in on a Monday morning that would change all that. It was from a family that lived on about eighty acres surrounded by national forest. I was never really sure what they did for a living, yet they seemed to get by and still be able to afford a few horses. A certain portion of the population in the Rocky Mountains has an uncanny knack for surviving without actually going to work every day, and the Linns were among this group.

Mr. Linn was a tall Abe Lincoln type, whose fashion statement never varied from a once-white T-shirt and an endless supply of dirty jeans. Much to my dismay, his wife was always impeccably dressed in what seemed to be the latest New York fashions. They made a unique pair: Mrs. Linn standing beside her shabby husband in her little black dress and designer shoes. They lived in a very modern log home on a little ranch, which would have been hard to maintain on Mr. Linn's woodcutting income. It was rumored that his wife was from a wealthy East Coast family and had moved to Colorado to find herself a mountain man. I did not doubt the validity of this gossip after observing her new Mercedes parked beside her husband's vintage pickup. However, I was invited there that day not to make judgments about their lifestyle but to check out a young horse that had had a hard weekend.

They had invited some friends up from the city that weekend for relaxation and horseback riding. Things were going well until the Linns asked their company to fetch one of the horses that was hiding in the pine trees about a mile from the house, since he would be needed if everyone was to have a mount. As the Linns explained it, Mr. Jeske, who was decked in shorts, black socks, and Rockports, directed his family to head out with pocketfuls of horse treats to entice the animal. But instead of riding horses out to find the missing creature, they opted to round him up with their oversized late-model SUV. Amazingly, they returned an hour later with the horse. Unfortunately, they had brought him back tied to the rear bumper of the vehicle. As you can imagine, this made for a less-than-happy animal. The Linns immediately realized that they should have given more detailed instructions for equine retrieval, but it was too late by then. Besides the mental damage, the horse had a few scrapes and small cuts that would need veterinary attention.

On my arrival, I found an extremely agitated patient, one who was not pleased to see yet another human appearing on the scene. He snorted and violently pulled back against the tree he was now tied to. His nostrils were flaring and he pawed the dirt, exposing roots that had never before seen daylight. It would take years on the couch to fix this one.

He wasn't a huge horse, but he made up for his size with quickness and tenacity. I didn't like the situation, yet I knew that the hair surrounding the wounds would have to be clipped and then the wounds thoroughly cleaned before I could leave. I retrieved a syringe and a sedative from the truck and went about the process of trying to insert the needle into the jugular vein in the horse's muscular, sweaty neck. As might be expected, the horse did not think that he needed to be sedated and proceeded to strike out with his front legs whenever I got near him with the syringe. I knew if I attempted to come in from the rear, he would kick out at me with both back legs. It was hard to blame him for not trusting humans after his ordeal behind the car, but it didn't change the fact that I needed to proceed with the treatment. After about twenty minutes, he decided to let me in close enough to gain access to the target area. The needle found its mark, and my thumb forced the plunger in with panic speed. In a few minutes, the medicine started to take effect, causing him to stumble a little, as if he'd had one too many. This was my cue to grab my clippers and get started with the treatment.

Usually, a tranquilized equine is not bothered by the quiet humming of cordless handheld clippers, but this particular steed was still hypersensitive and sprang back to complete consciousness as I began to work. He managed to rear up, placing his right knee between my legs as he went. It is not hard to imagine which of my body parts the knee connected with. I found myself lying on the ground eight feet away from where I had been standing a half second before. An unearthly pain began to crawl up my pelvis and abdomen. It was the same sensation I remember having on the playground when one of my classmates missed the soccer ball and landed his foot in my crotch instead, except this blow came from a nine-hundred-pound horse, not a one-hundred-pound sixth grader. The effect was tenfold, causing me to writhe on rough, decomposed granite in a fetal position.

The clippers I was holding had flown out of my hand and hit a nearby tree, fracturing into multiple pieces. As I began to regain my senses, it became apparent that Mr. Linn was fighting with the horse to keep him from coming after me again. The animal's ears were pressed flat against the back of his head, his teeth were bared, and the conjunctiva around his eyes was bright red with anger. It was hard to believe that this animal had such a vendetta for me, but he was determined that no human was going to mess with him again.

Working to hold on to a shred of dignity, I was able to get to my feet. Still doubled over and walking very stiffly, I gathered up the remains of my clippers in the hope of salvaging some functional parts. The truck seemed as if it were miles away, but I was able to get to it at a snail's pace. Clinging to it for support, I dug out some ointment for the Linns to apply to the horse's wounds themselves and some antibiotic powder to put in his food. I managed to drive home, although I felt every bump along the way as if it were a land mine.

After two days, I could finally stand up almost straight and had worked up the courage to go back to work, albeit loaded up on Advil. Unfortunately, most small veterinary clinics don't offer sick or personal days; besides, I didn't want to have to explain to a lot of clients which injured body part was causing me to miss work. The next couple of weeks, I was definitely more cautious on horse calls.

Since then, trying to stay out of the line of fire while keeping my legs close together has prevented a repeat performance, but every time I see that crazed, wild-eyed look in a horse, this experience replays in my brain. It takes only a split second for an animal this largé to do irreparable damage to a human being. I was lucky to get off with just a warning and not a disabling injury. It's natural for frightened animals to protect themselves, and you can't blame them for doing so. But I have to say that this rationale doesn't make it hurt any less.

Taking the Bait

Sometimes we humans are not the most intelligent creatures, and occasionally we even involve animals in our stupidity. In veterinary practice, it seems like these lapses in judgment occur most often on holiday weekends. Here in the West, people who live anywhere within a ten-hour radius of the mountains will load up every possession they might need for a lunar landing, dust off the camper trailer, and head for the high country. Unfortunately, the list of essential camping gear often involves an unsuspecting pet. I always dread these weekends because animals from the suburban environment so often seem to find trouble in the mountains.

On one particular Saturday morning of a Fourth of July weekend, we got a call from a beer, bait, and gas shop in a lake resort area about twenty miles from the clinic. The lake, a tranquil body of water surrounded by shimmering peaks, was usually a haven for wildlife and the occasional local fisherman, but on summer weekends it was transformed into a refugee camp. I have often wondered how much fun it can be to get away to a place where one family is practically on top of another. It seems a lot like some of the neighborhoods the people are escaping from. I heard Lorraine, our receptionist, sigh as she got off the phone that morning. "Tourists! They've had some trouble with their cat and are on their way in. They were so upset, that was all the information I could get out of them."

After the phone call, we continued with those clients who had scheduled appointments. Saturday mornings in veterinary clinics are always a little crazy because most people are off work and have time to bring in their pets. As expected, we already had a full waiting room that morning. The white plastic chairs that lined the walls were all occupied with impatient clients. An older man held a thin gray miniature poodle, whose breath desecrated the entire room, as if something had died in its mouth. A teenage girl sat with an immense mastiff at her feet, the dog sprawling on the yellow linoleum. Duke, the mastiff, was in for his biannual toenail trim, which always involved several helpers and looked something like a professional wrestling extravaganza. Another woman sat in the corner clutching her terrified cat, who would periodically retch as if trying to vomit, yet nothing came out. I was certain that at any minute a hair ball would eject from the feline's mouth and shoot across the room. The other seats were taken by those with pets in need of routine vaccinations and exams.

I was in the middle of explaining canine dental care to the fire-breathing poodle's owner when our injured cat and his owners burst through the door. The wounded cat had not fallen prey to any creature of the forest but was presented with a long strand of fishing line hanging from its mouth and a look of terror in its eyes. The young couple whom the cat belonged to had, for some reason, decided to take the pet fishing for the weekend. Usually, members of the feline species are not considered the best companions for outdoor activities, since they prefer the plush surroundings of home or a dogproof yard. I don't know if these relative newlyweds felt bad about leaving the cat at home or if it substituted for the child they did not yet have. Whatever the reason, the plan turned out to be a less-than-perfect one.

The Shaws looked to be in their late twenties and not very much like the outdoorsy type. Brad, a little doughy and pale, was wearing a pair of Hawaiian shorts and a T-shirt with the Greek letters of a fraternity on the front. His wife, Brenda, had shiny white skin that reeked of sunscreen. She hardly seemed old enough to be married, yet she appeared to be the chief of this family unit. "Please help us—we called ahead," she choked out between breaths. I wanted to make a joke about having held a table for three, but I deemed this not to be the appropriate time, given their frightened looks. The little cat was completely freaked-out.

Brenda quickly explained that they had been using bright red salmon eggs for fishing bait, and when Brad drew back to cast, Socks had not been able to resist swallowing the entire bait and hook. The round red eggs dangling at the end of a fishing line must have looked to Socks like an elaborate cat toy. "We tried to get it out," she cried, "but Socks freaked." So they had cut the line free and headed our way with the hook still inside the cat.

Driving for thirty minutes with Socks attempting to get air in past a fishhook must have seemed like being in a cage with a grizzly bear. Brad had taken the brunt of the attack. He'd had the task of holding the frightened feline on the trip in. His thighs and hands looked as if they had been through a paper shredder. Blood seeped from the multitude of bite wounds, and his hands had begun to swell.

I grabbed the cat away from Brad's stiff hands and placed him on the exam table. Christie already had a syringeful of anesthetic drawn up, and I slid it into the muscle of the cat's rear leg. The injection was unnoticed by the cat, whose attention was completely on the pesky fishhook. In just a few minutes, sleep overwhelmed him, finally bringing peace to the entire office. The anesthesia allowed us to get a small hemostat through the cat's mouth and down to the hook. With some gentle twisting, the hook came loose, and Socks could breathe easy again. He received an antiinflammatory injection to reduce the swelling in his throat, and Christie placed him in a recovery cage in the back. The short-acting anesthetic quickly wore off, and the feline was soon acting as if nothing had happened.

Within an hour, Socks was purring and looking for food. The humans, unfortunately, were not faring as well. By the time I walked back into the waiting room to give them the good news about Socks, Brad's hands looked like catchers' mitts. The signs indicated infection was beginning to brew. Cats normally carry a lot of bacteria on their teeth and claws, so unsuspecting victims almost always end up with an infection. Left untreated, these injuries can even be fatal.

We instructed Brad that he had to see a physician immediately, but, like most of us men, he went the macho route, brushing off his condition as "no big deal." Finally, after much nagging by Brenda and me, in addition to even more swelling, he caved in. They collected a much-relieved Socks, paid the bill, and headed for a local

M.D. I was sure this time the story of how the injuries came about would be even more embarrassing for the beleaguered couple.

After they left, we went on with the day, working through the rest of our Saturday patients and trying to resist the urge to make catfish jokes.

Miniature Menace

Animals, like people, should never be underestimated due to their size. Some of the toughest dogs I've dealt with have weighed under thirty pounds. The average ten-pound cat can wreak havoc if asked to do something that might seem even slightly inappropriate in feline society. But Jefferson, a Sicilian donkey, has been a standout in my career as a representative of the "small but mighty" crowd. Sicilian donkeys are actually a miniature version of their larger counterparts, with which most of us are familiar. Like the rest of the occupants of the island for which they are named, these long-eared Sicilians are not to be slighted. The little burros are very cute at first glance. They have a wiry gray or black coat and tiny dark hooves as hard as graphite. They usually stand about two and a half feet at the shoulder and are dominated by a huge set of fuzzy sound detectors. Not many predators are quiet enough to sneak into their space without being noticed.

My neighbor has an unneutered male named Arnold, but some-one forgot to tell him that he's a miniature. He struts around the horses that he shares the pasture with as if he were the big man on campus, and he has a set of lungs that Pavarotti would have been proud of. Every day when my neighbor turns on the house lights at 5:30 A.M., the little fellow lets go, braying at least ten times, remind-ing his owner that he will need to be fed soon and acting as an alarm clock for the entire neighborhood in the process. Fortunately, on weekends my neighbor tends to sleep in, not flipping the lights on until seven. After hearing the early morning wake-up call, people are always taken aback when they actually meet the perpetrator. They expect a beast that can at least look over the top wire on the fence.

My client Jefferson was not much different from my neighbor's donkey—maybe even a little more belligerent and cocky. He also lived with a pastureful of horses and filled the role of leader when-ever the opportunity arose. His owners may have spoiled him just a little, as he had gotten very hard to handle over the previous couple of years. He would hear my truck pull in the driveway and begin to plan his getaway. Even when it came to vaccinations or routine treat-ments, he would practically have to be lashed to a post just to slow him down long enough to accomplish my task.

Jefferson led a life of significant excess, and his diet had never been restricted. Out of love, he had been fed a regular diet of horse treats and carrots on top of his normal hay rations, and as a conse-quence he had become nearly as wide as he was tall. In fact, his back had gotten so wide, you could easily have served a meal for four on it. I talked to the Murphys many times about Jefferson's weight issues, but Mrs. Murphy could never resist his sad brown eyes and the long, batting lashes. All she ever said was, "He's just so darn cute, I can't deprive him of anything."

Although I was never sure who owned whom, Mrs. Murphy clearly loved Jefferson. She was a cheery forty-year-old who was always in great physical condition. She rode her mountain bike religiously every day and ate only the healthiest of foods. Yet none of these habits seemed to trickle down to Jefferson. I always wanted to suggest she take him with her on a few bike rides, but I couldn't quite get myself to bring it up. His attitude also showed some parallels to that of a spoiled child who always gets what he or she wants. Jefferson was never forced to do anything he didn't want to do. But on this particular visit, I finally decided I would have to change that mind-set.

I was called because Jefferson had a front leg full of porcupine quills as a result of having attempted to stomp on the small but well-protected animal. The quills would migrate into Jefferson's tendons and joints if not removed rather quickly. With Mrs. Murphy gone for this midsummer weekend, her husband, Don, and I were left to talk Jefferson into the procedure. Luckily, Don was a strong fellow who was in good shape, because Jefferson and his comrades had full run of a twenty-acre pasture, with no barn or catch pen to coax him into. This meant that we would have to corner the little monster and get a halter on him.

I knew that this was going to be a much larger job than it might have seemed to the casual observer, especially with Jefferson's buddy and bodyguard protecting him. A big sorrel draft horse named Ed had decided that his position in life was to watch over Jefferson, keeping him safe from husbands and veterinarians. The little donkey would run in and out of Ed's legs as they moved across the field together. If we got too close, Ed would lay back his ears and bare his teeth to keep us at bay. Finally, Jefferson made a wrong step, allowing Don to get between him and Ed. Working together, we drove the tough little guy into an area where the sides of the fence came together, forming a corner. We moved in slowly while Jefferson nervously tried to find an escape route. He attempted to dart past us as his world got smaller bit by bit. We almost had him, but then he decided that I was the weakest link and made his move to run past me. I stuck out my arm with the intention of hooking him in the crook of my elbow, but I had drastically underestimated him. Jefferson had played this game before, and he became airborne just as his chest connected with my arm. From afar, the scene must have unfolded like an old cartoon. He knocked my 235 pounds easily onto the ground and stormed away. It was not a stretch to believe he was laughing at me with his head held high as he returned to his comrades. Don was laughing, too. "Doc," he said, "he ran you over as if you weren't even there. It's a good thing he's only a miniature."

If there was any doubt what we were up to before, the donkey had now broken the code and the secret was out. The second try would be even harder. By the time Don and I had caught our breath and gathered some strength back, Jefferson was hiding directly under his guardian. Ed's tree-trunk legs stood like pillars to hold back intruders. After twenty more minutes of darting, dodging, and near-death experiences with Ed, we got them apart again. With Jefferson back in the corner, we began to close the trap once more. This attempt would have to be different, because both humans were starting to lose steam, while our prey was no worse for wear.

I have to admit to feeling great relief when the determined little donkey turned toward Don and made a run for it. Learning from my shortcomings, Don decided to go for a tackle. But this was no high school football player from a quarter century ago, and there were no penalties for use of teeth or hoof. I'll give Don credit for agility and strength, but not for self-preservation. He got a hold of the quill-carrying running back and was dragged well past the goal line. Still holding on for dear life, Don somehow managed to get Jefferson onto his side. I came sprinting in from the side with a halter and jumped onto the pile.

Just after Jefferson hit the ground, he began to thrash Don relentlessly with both back legs. As I struggled with the halter, I could see Don's face redden and grimace from the pain. Then, as I was about to fasten the halter in place, I felt a crushing pain in my left hand. No, it wasn't a heart attack—my entire hand was in Jefferson's mouth, and his incisors were clamped down on it like a vise. I managed to yank it out of his grip, tearing the skin as I did so. Warm blood ran down my arm, and I was about to give in when I realized Don was still taking a beating. As I finished my job of locking the halter on tight, Don and I let our patient up and gasped for breath, both of us bent over, our hands on our knees, sucking at the thin mountain air for its precious oxygen.

Jefferson let us recover in the spirit of fair play, but when I pulled out the hemostats for quill removal, he tried another break for safety. No way would we let him go this time. Don held on to the lead rope and I went for the quills, removing them quickly as Jefferson reared and kicked. Fortunately, I was used to moving targets during this type of procedure, and it was over in minutes. I might have been disappointed if he had not taken that last shot at us with both back legs when we let him go. I like to think it was his version of a thank-you, but I'm afraid he meant something a little different. At least the quills were no longer in his leg, and no infection or lameness would ensue.

Don limped back to the house, with me dragging behind, nursing my hand. His pants were torn in several places and bruises were starting to form where the flesh showed through. "If only we could have convinced him it was for his own good," he mumbled. "That would have made it a lot easier." I nodded in agreement and suggested that he needed some corral facilities in case there was a next time.

A week later, I saw Don at the lumberyard, buying supplies for a new barn and pens. "I started thinking about what you said the other day, about there being a next time," he explained. "I realized you might be a little harder to get hold of if we had another veterinary emergency with Jefferson. So I'm starting the project this weekend." He hesitated, then spoke again. "Besides, my wife spotted another porcupine in the pasture this morning."

Who's the Boss?

Although most veterinary clinics have an owner or at least an office manager, the real boss doesn't have a name on the sign out front, a big office, or a lot of framed certificates on the wall. But the real boss does get a private litter box.

Just about every practice has a mascot cat, and these lucky animals always act as if they are running the show. The feline in charge will often strut, tail straight in the air, through the exam room to check out the quality of patient care or leap onto the operating table to ruin the sterile surgery area. If the waiting room is filled with lowly canines, the cat may peruse the area, testing the strength of owners and their leashes. If bored with harassing the patrons, the feline will assume a supervisory position on the reception counter. This allows the animal to take on a public-relations role as well by generously giving human clients the opportunity to caress it while paying their bills.

The application for clinic cat is not a simple one. Most find their way into this position because they were strays that no one wanted or hard-luck cases that needed expensive medical treatment, and no one returned to pick them up. No matter how they end up at the office, they will eventually win the hearts of the humans and climb the corporate ladder quickly.

My favorite boss cat was a beautiful gray tabby appropriately named Beastie Cat. She was found on the crest of a nearby mountain pass, scrounging out an existence for herself and seven kittens. They were probably dumped off by someone who was disappointed when one feline pet became eight. This above-timberline environment was no place to be raising a family; small rodent meals were scarce and so was shelter, not to mention an abundance of wind, cold, and lightning storms. But Beastie Cat must have been quite a mountaineer and an innovative hunter because she and her family fared pretty well.

My boss was out on a Jeep ride when he stumbled upon the feline family, and they were more than willing to jump in with him. On their arrival at the clinic, they were treated as if they had checked into the spa at the Ritz. Everybody was bathed, brushed, and de-wormed. Next they were treated to a daily buffet of gourmet cat food, and within two weeks, all signs of a tough lifestyle had fallen away. They were given full run of the clinic, which became a rumpus room for the kittens. Sliding across the linoleum floors and holding "fur ball" wrestling meets provided hours of entertainment for all of us. Christie didn't enjoy their antics as much as the rest of us, since she got the job of maintaining the litter box, a task that got bigger by the day. As she said, with a scoop in one hand, "All they do is eat and . . ." Beastie Cat was not that amused with her kittens' rambunctious behavior, either. She spent exhausting days attempting to keep some kind of order within her brood, a losing proposition for even the best of feline families.

The day came when it was time to find the kittens new homes. They easily found cozy casas with great clients, but their mom was not so lucky, although it's true she had a few traits that made her a less-than-perfect house pet. Physically, she was fine; her problems were definitely more psychological. We would often find her lying on her back in the middle of the clinic driveway, feet straight up in the air. By some miracle, she never got run over. Sometimes she got along with the other animals that came through the door and sometimes she didn't. If she didn't care for a patient, she would welcome the animal at the door by hissing and spitting, as if to say, How dare you disturb me, even if you do have a life-threatening injury? Occasionally, a curious dog would get too close and get a razor-sharp claw across the snout. Owners never seemed to see the humor in their puppy leaving the office with a nose full of sutures when he was there only for a rabies vaccination. We never ruled out the possibility that she was demonically possessed; nor was an exorcism considered out of the question. She was a little bit of a liability, but she was always entertaining, and besides, no one else would have her. Some days, her mental illness actually seemed to be cured. She would be friendly, personable, and affectionate. Then the next day, her attitude might be closer to that of a mountain lion with a migraine.

Beastie not only targeted clients and patients; the staff was not immune to her bad-hair days, either. It was not uncommon for her to bite one of us for no reason at all or lash out at our hands with her paw while we were writing out a prescription. At one point, she developed an ear infection and was less than happy about having her ear canal irrigated. The next morning, I didn't notice the thank-you gift she had left for me on my chair until it was too late. An unfamiliar feeling against my jeans and then the very familiar odor of cat feces let me know she had reaped her vengeance. How do you get back at a cat for that?

My most memorable Beastie Cat experience occurred on a lazy July Sunday afternoon. I was on the couch, in the middle of watching one of those coming-of-age TV movies that I had seen at least five times before. I still had the same television that my roommate and I had bought in college for twelve dollars—one of those with a lot of wood and large cloth-covered speakers on each side. The movie was just about to put me to sleep when my pager threw a curve in my afternoon. I returned the call, only to find that there would be no nap that day.

"Our German shepherd jumped off the deck to chase a squirrel, and now he won't put any weight on his front left leg. Can you take a look at him?" Mr. Miller asked. I could tell from his voice that he had been hoping my boss would be the one to call him back, but I would have to do on short notice. They would meet me at the clinic in five minutes, and I was dreading it. I pulled into the driveway and was hit by that familiar smell of pine produced by the old-growth ponderosa that surrounded the perimeter of the building. The forty-foot giants seemed to take away some of the stress and sterility from the veterinary hospital atmosphere.

The Millers were nice enough, but their kids were out of control. Mr. Miller was a quiet, hardworking man of about forty-five, with graying hair and a perpetually exhausted appearance. Mrs. Miller was very similar in female form, except she appeared even more worn-out than her mate. The five children—all loud, spoiled, and completely devoid of manners—were making their parents' lives a living hell. The kids ranged in age from about four to fifteen, and the entire brood was running around the building, rattling door-knobs, when I got to the clinic that day.

Mrs. Miller finally yelled out from their old Subaru wagon, "Come on, kids. If you're not good, we won't let you watch if there's any blood involved." Even though it sounded like a good argument, especially for this crew of miscreants, the "Brady Bunch" continued to attempt their break-in. I wanted to pull back out of the driveway and hotfoot it back to my cabin, but I had to get it together for the dog's sake. After managing to unlock the door amid the chaos, I stood back as the entire family flooded into the waiting room. Mr. Miller and I carried the big dog into the exam room and eased him onto the Formica exam table.

My examination of the leg elicited a yelp when I flexed the carpal joint above the paw. I informed the spectators that I needed to take an X ray, and they all nodded their approval. Even the four-year-old gave me the okay. Mr. Miller helped me get Scout into the radiology area and then went back out with the rest of the pack to avoid radiation exposure. After strapping on the fashionable lead apron and matching gloves, I talked Scout into allowing me to snap a couple of different views. This was all taking some time, and I could sense the natives getting a little restless in the next room. By the time the films were soaked in developing chemicals, the children were bouncing around the clinic as if it were one of those inflatable castles that people rent for birthday parties. They had opened every door, helped themselves to the bandage materials, and removed my diploma from the wall to determine whether or not I was qualified to be treating their pet. The parents had obviously given up on discipline and looked like they were longing for the days of life without offspring. The Millers were elated to hear that Scout had no fractures and could go home with just a support wrap. They were also very relieved to avoid the expense of surgery.

Meanwhile, the reform-school candidates had moved back into the waiting room, and the noise level was reaching an all-time high. But despite the racket, I could suddenly hear a low, deep growl from behind the counter. Beastie Cat had been napping on the reception- ist's chair the entire time, and now she was awake. As I strode down the short hallway, I felt as if I were moving in slow motion. I tried to reach the waiting room before the inevitable happened, but I was too late. There was a serpentlike hiss, followed by a scream and a stam- pede of footsteps out the door. All I witnessed by the time I arrived were a few drops of human blood on the floor and a triumphant fe- line whipping her tail as if to invite a rematch. Mrs. Miller, the only family member still in the building, stood back from the counter, holding her open checkbook.

It took all my strength to hold back laughter as I wrote up the bill. I was fully expecting a comment about our ill-mannered kitty, but it didn't happen. Mrs. Miller thanked me profusely. "We really appre- ciate your taking care of old Scout," she said. "We weren't sure about you at first, but now we feel comfortable with you if no one else is available." I didn't allow myself to think of an appropriate response to that. As they drove away, I could see the children all sitting quietly in the old car. Beastie had accomplished what the parents could not.

Two weeks later, they brought Scout back in for a recheck. The family filed in one by one and sat silently in the plastic chairs. Beastie Cat lay on the counter, staring them down while slapping her tail rhythmically against the surface, but no one challenged her. I appre- ciated that cat a lot more from then on. In fact, I even learned to overlook most of her psychotic episodes.

Slap Shot

One of my favorite places to make a house call is a guest ranch tucked into the Rockies beside a beautiful mountain river. The ranch consists of a main lodge with outlying stone and log buildings with views of snowy peaks. The owners keep seventy horses of every color, age, and breed. People come from all around the world to stay at the ranch and trail-ride for a week at a time. With this many animals, the ranch keeps me busy, especially during the summer months. On one particular day, the horses, who were getting the week off, needed some routine maintenance. So Christie brushed the crumbs from my previous day's lunch off the passenger seat of the pickup, shook her head at me, and crawled in for our ride to the guest ranch.

As I steered the truck out of the driveway and onto the risky mountain highway, Christie started organizing the paperwork on my dash. I always had a mess of receipts on my dash, but it had never seemed to bother her before. She was abnormally quiet that morning, and I had a feeling I knew what the problem might be related to. Christie had met a guy about a month before and was very excited about this one. I had met him briefly at the clinic—too brief an encounter to make a proper judgment, I admit, but I've never trusted men with excessive jewelry.

After ten minutes of Christie's paper shuffling, my urge to plunge into dangerous territory overwhelmed me. "So . . . how was your weekend?" I asked. No response; we sat in uncomfortable silence for the next couple of minutes.

Finally, she spoke, eyes still focused out the window. "Men suck!"

Oh boy, I thought, now I've opened the can. "Okay, what happened?"

She stared down at her lap. "I mentioned that my parents wanted to have us over for supper," she began, "and he gave me the 'Maybe we should date other people' talk. Then he moved onto his 'I'm not looking for a long-term relationship' finale."

I wondered what I should say. I wasn't surprised that this had happened. Most guys considered those lines to be standard fare, not that I would have known, since I hadn't had a date in months. The best I could come up with was, "Well, maybe it's for the best." This just got me an icy glare and more silence, but she needed to talk to someone about it, so that didn't last too long. She went on about how she had thought this might be "the guy" and how much they had in common. Having heard this all before from her about other guys, I decided it would be safest just to nod my head and throw in an occasional "Uh-huh." At last, we pulled off the highway and down the windy gravel road into the guest ranch.

Four horses were tied to the hitching rail just outside the barn, where the saddles and tack were kept. At the sound of our truck, an overdressed twenty-something wrangler strode out of the barn. He had on the classic black felt cowboy hat and tight jeans. His shirt had ivory buttons and a yoke design on the front and back. But the clothes were pressed and new, not well used like those of someone who was working hard. He was obviously very proud of his outfit and shoved out his chest when he saw Christie get out of the truck.

He stuck out his hand to me. "I'm Shane, from Fort Worth. Got lots of experience with horses. Back home, we wouldn't have hired a vet to do this; we'd have done it ourselves." I was starting to see why Shane had been left behind to "help us," instead of taking people out for rides with the others.

The first three horses had sharp points on their back teeth that needed to be filed off so they could chew better. This procedure is known as "teeth floating." As we worked down the row, I was amused by Shane's attempts to flirt with Christie. Of course, she completely ignored his overtures, to the point that I was actually getting a little embarrassed for him. The last equine was having some trouble urinating and needed to have his sheath cleaned. I gave him some sedation to make the procedure safer and easier, then waited patiently for it to take effect, trying at the same time to distract Shane from Christie by making small talk about Texas.

After a few minutes, the sedation started to kick in, and the horse's head began to drop. The other side effect of the sedative was that the part that needed to be cleaned dropped down also. This situation would usually have been accompanied by a few marginal jokes and snickers, but that day the audience reaction could not have come at a more inappropriate time. Shane cleared his throat. All I could think was, Oh, no, please don't, but here it came anyway. He leaned against the horse with one arm, crossed his legs, and said in his best Texas drawl, "Well, you know, this horse doesn't have anything on me."

I turned immediately toward Christie. Her face was beet red, not with embarrassment but anger. She was completely fed up with men, and this poor excuse for one had put her over the edge. Her blue eyes narrowed into demonic slits, and her face contorted into a shape I hadn't seen before. She cut loose on him with expletives not to be repeated, then sent him off with his tail between his legs. I debated about calling the insurance company right then to discuss liability coverage or waiting to see how things panned out. We finished our work in silence and without Shane.

On our way back to the clinic, Christie's tough exterior started to melt away, and as she softened, the tears began to come. "I'm sorry, I never should have reacted that way, but that guy was being such a jerk," she squeaked out between the tears.

Searching for the right words, the best I could come up with was, "Well, you've just got a lot going on today, don't you think?" She nodded and we continued down the highway, laughing about Shane's obvious insecurities, not to mention his complete lack of taste.

It was only about a week after the "Men suck" incident that I had to return to the ranch for an evening emergency. That night, an animal dealt out the punishment to an unsuspecting Shane that Christie would have liked to give him.

This particular summer evening, I was called to the ranch to treat a horse with a bellyache. A sweet young woman from Georgia came out to the corral to help me. She filled me in on the animal's symptoms, and we agreed that colic was the problem. Colic in horses is usually caused by some form of blockage in the intestine and makes them extremely uncomfortable, since they cannot vomit. This poor horse was no exception, and we both just wanted to make him feel better. I placed a plastic tube through the patient's nose and down to the stomach, then pumped mineral oil through the tube to help get his bowels moving. After that, I gave him an injection of painkiller, and within a few minutes the horse started looking for something to eat.

I was packing to leave when a couple of the male employees came out of the lodge, moving in the direction of the burro pen. The two burros were named Lefty and Poncho. They were a mangy pair, with long shaggy hair that hung over their eyes and broomlike tails that would whip back and forth when they were upset. Burros are not large animals, but they are extremely strong for their size. They have a low center of gravity and are very hard to hang on to if they decide not to cooperate. These two were especially tough, since they had been wild originally and then had been brought in from the desert a few years before as part of a rescue effort.

As the two young men moved across in front of us in the last of the day's sunlight, I recognized one of them as Shane. His confidence had been built back up by that time and been helped by the beers he'd had with supper. He had decided to attempt to ride Lefty. This was entertainment I could not resist getting a good seat for, since Lefty had never been ridden. One might have been tempted to worry about Lefty's well-being, but this would have been a concern only if you hadn't been around burros.

The slightly tipsy wanna-be cowboy hauled himself over the corral fence, grabbed a halter, and headed for Lefty. He got the halter on the burro's head and attached a lead rope to it. Then, with a boost from his cohort, he was on Lefty's back. He let out a "Yee ha!" and then the games began. The second Shane's butt and Lefty's back made contact, Lefty leaped straight up, all four feet off the ground, as if he were jet-propelled. I could see at least three feet of light between rider and beast before they slammed to earth for the second round. Lefty had barely touched down before he kicked both back legs into the air and shot his rider toward the stars. Shane might have been willing to call it quits at that point, except for the fact that Lefty wasn't done with him yet. As only a burro could, Lefty regrouped and kicked Shane in the groin on his way back to earth.

In a matter of seconds, the burro had completely debilitated his human challenger and was back to munching on hay as if nothing had happened. The young wrangler lay moaning in a pile of donkey manure as I headed toward my pickup. I understand that he didn't boast about anything the rest of the summer.

The next time I saw Shane was about a week later, and he still wasn't walking right. He moved as if he were trying to hold a bowling ball between his legs. The rest of the staff said he hadn't been even close to getting back on a horse since his dance with Lefty. I can't imagine what hours in a saddle would have felt like to a man in his condition.

Christie seemed to think his predicament was quite humorous. She did deserve her revenge, but as a fellow Y chromosome holder, I couldn't help feeling a little sorry for him. I guess you could call it "sympathy pain."

Attention Deficit

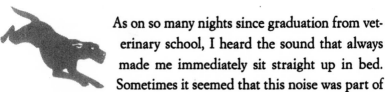As on so many nights since graduation from vet-
erinary school, I heard the sound that always
made me immediately sit straight up in bed.
Sometimes it seemed that this noise was part of
a dream—a fire alarm or a school bell telling me I was late for class.
After shaking off the dream that night, I was hit by the harsh reality
that it was my pager and that I would probably have to get out of bed
and take off into the night. At the very least, I would have to wake
myself up enough to call these people back and act completely prepared to deal with whatever four-legged emergency they had.

Just as on so many nights before, I picked up the phone beside my
bed and called my voice mail to retrieve the message. Then, while
struggling to keep my eyes open, I dialed the number that was given.
After about eight rings, a sleepy male voice on the other end an-
swered. Explaining that I was Dr. Wells, returning his call about the
sick dog, I was met by a brief silence, followed by some expletives

about how late it was and the slamming down of the phone. Now I was really awake.

Dialing the correct number this time, I reached Mrs. Feller, who explained that her new shih tzu puppy, Hercules, was practically unconscious and needed to be seen right away. Her voice was shaky, nearly breaking down into a full-blown cry. I told her to head for the clinic and that I would meet her there. Pulling on my clothes, I went out into the night to warm up my truck, then drove, bleary-eyed, to the clinic—a route so familiar that the vehicle seemed to maneuver it on its own.

By the time I reached the clinic, Mrs. Feller was already sitting in the parking lot. She was a well-dressed, soccer mom type, accessorized with the appropriate battleship SUV. Standing on the clinic's wooden deck with her, I rifled through my keys, trying three different ones before finding the one that worked. Mrs. Feller watched me anxiously, waiting to get her ailing puppy inside for treatment. Finally getting the door open, I fumbled in the dark for the light switch to bring the clinic to life.

At last we were in the exam room, and Mrs. Feller placed the small and nearly comatose pup on the exam table. The poor little guy was nothing but fur-covered bones as he lay there on the cold Formica tabletop, his chest rising slowly with every labored breath. I stared down at him with a sickening feeling in my stomach. I had no idea what to do next—not an uncommon response for a young veterinarian to have. There was no sign of trauma or fever to indicate an infection. His heart and lungs also sounded normal. Sweat was beginning to run down my nose.

Mrs. Feller began to pick up on my lack of a diagnosis. "Do you have any idea what is wrong with him?" she asked, obviously getting a little nervous about my abilities. I ignored her doubt for the moment and began asking her all the appropriate questions: Was there something Hercules could have eaten from the garbage? Would anyone have had a reason to poison him? As I continued to try to pry something helpful from the puppy's history, I noticed Mrs. Feller start to fidget a little. She wouldn't look at me, staring only at the lifeless little dog. It seemed as if she had something to say but couldn't quite get it out.

Eventually, I stopped asking questions, giving her the opportunity to speak. After about a minute, she said, "I took Hercules to another veterinary clinic earlier in the week for a diarrhea problem. They prescribed some medicine for an intestinal parasite, so I picked it up at a local pharmacy that afternoon." She hadn't wanted to tell me this because she'd been afraid I wouldn't see her dog if I had known that we were not her regular veterinarians. Of course, the other clinic did not handle after-hours emergencies.

After fessing up, she began to tell me about how they had moved from California the previous year with their first shih tzu, Spike. Not long after arriving in the Rocky Mountains, they'd let Spike out to do his routine business. But on that particular November evening, the first snow of the season was falling hard. Unfortunately, neither Spike nor his family was very familiar with mountain snowstorms, and Spike never returned to the house. Tears filled Mrs. Feller's eyes as she explained how they found Spike the following spring. He had been near a favorite spot next to the curb when the snowplow had come by. I realized that this had been quite a stress on the family, and now the dog they had gotten to replace Spike was deteriorating right in front of me.

"Is there anything else you can think of that might have triggered his illness?" I asked hopefully.

She gave it one more try. "Well, you know, he didn't really start going downhill until I started the intestinal treatment." She dumped her purse out onto the table, and an amber pill bottle rolled free of the other contents.

A close study of the bottle showed these to be the appropriate tablets, but the dosage seemed a little high. I excused myself and headed for the back of the clinic to check the drug formulary. I didn't want her to realize that I didn't know the exact dose of every possible pharmaceutical for every size of dog. To my astonishment, Hercules had been getting the correct dose—for an adult Saint Bernard. Not having much experience with this kind of overdose, I decided it would be best to contact Poison Control.

The expert on call yawned as she looked up the treatment for this specific toxicity. "How much did you say that the pup was getting?" When I gave her the numbers, I heard a little gasp on the other end of the line. "I have never heard of an overdose that large for this medication," she said, sounding very much awake.

After these discouraging words, I followed her instructions for treatment. IV fluids seemed to be the main component of the protocol, so I dug out the smallest catheter that I could find and shaved Hercules' left front leg to accentuate the cephalic vein. No magic cure or foolproof antidote was available, just fluids to accelerate the drug's elimination through the puppy's kidneys. Getting an IV catheter into his tiny vein was like threading a python through the eye of a needle. In addition to the blood vessel being small to begin with, the pup was severely dehydrated, which further decreased the diameter of the vein. After poking and prodding for several very tense minutes, with Mrs. Feller glaring over my shoulder, I gave up on getting the catheter placed in that vein. At this point, I thought I heard her mumble something about how long I had been out of school. Fortunately, dogs have two front legs, and luck was with me on the right front one. With everything ready to go, I hooked up a bag of fluids and put Hercules on a heated pad in one of the stainless-steal kennels. Now it was out of our hands; I just hoped it wasn't too late.

I discussed the less-than-favorable prognosis with Mrs. Feller, and she went home for what remained of the night, leaving me alone with the little patient. The fluid dripped in very slowly—if the solution is run in too quickly, a dog's lungs will fill with fluid, so patience is a virtue. Pulling up the most comfortable office chair we had, I began to settle in. Sleep quickly started to become harder to fight, and I drifted in and out, occasionally waking up just long enough to check on Hercules' condition.

I had no idea how much time had passed when the shrill yipping of a very upset little dog woke me suddenly. Rubbing the sleep out of my eyes, I could see the sun peeking through the small window beside the kennels in the back room of the clinic, where Hercules and I had spent the night. The plastic clock on the wall read 6:00 A.M. It took me a moment to realize that the persistent barking was coming from Hercules.

He was bouncing around in the cage, tangled up in the IV tubing and looking for food. His little eyes were bright, and his pink tongue was wagging in happiness. I got up out of my chair and found myself standing in a pool of dog urine. It was all that was left of the overdose. This was one of the few times I was happy about standing in such a puddle. As I filled Hercules' dog dish, he nearly took off my finger to get to the food. Mrs. Feller was elated when I called her with the good news, and she couldn't get off the phone fast enough to come pick him up.

It is easy to make this kind of a call, especially when there has been a good chance things could have gone the other way. Making phone calls to convey the opposite outcome is one of my least favorite responsibilities of veterinary practice. Curing an animal that is very ill gives one a great deal of satisfaction. I especially look forward to seeing such patients again for routine visits to follow their progress after these kinds of serious ordeals, but I never saw Hercules again. Mrs. Feller explained to Christie that she would rather see an older, more experienced practitioner, and she returned to her previous veterinarian for Hercules' future care.

Yak Attack

As a rule, the closer it is to sundown, the less chance there is that someone will call with an emergency. People tend not to notice their outdoor pets again until morning, but on one particular summer night, I didn't quite make it. The pager began buzzing and jumping around on the coffee table in front of the television about 8:00 P.M. It was one of those times that I hoped I was just imagining it. I sat staring at the pager until it went off again a few minutes later, confirming the worst. I'd been caught off guard, falsely comfortable in the hope that I was settled in for the night. Oh, to have one night of peace. Reluctantly, I dialed the number, then waited. On the sixth ring, a woman said, "Hello." "Yes, this is Dr. Wells returning your call," I replied. "Oh, yes, thank you for calling back. We just talked to two other veterinarians, but they don't work on yaks," she informed me. "I'm sorry, did you say yaks?" I asked, assuming that I had not heard her correctly. "Yes, I said yaks, Tibetan yaks. Do you work on them? We have one that is not doing well at all." I knew that this would be my chance to get out of this call. I had been down similar roads before, and all it would have taken was a simple no. I could have hung up and watched the evening news. Yet there was an animal in trouble, and even though I had seen yaks only in zoos, how much different could they be from a cow? I gave her my answer: "I guess this will be the first time." She seemed happy that I was willing to give it a try, and she gave me directions on how to get to their place.

When called out after hours, you sometimes really have to force yourself to get out of the chair and just keep moving forward. I jammed my feet back into my smelly boots and tugged on the laces, snapping one off in my hand. After tying my shoestrings back together, I got out the door, armed with the directions and a complete lack of knowledge in yak medicine. The route took me past many familiar roads, then eventually down a fairly obscure one, which was new to me. Darkness was chasing me as the curves and landmarks became harder to make out. The address was painted on a board nailed to a tree beside the driveway. The driveway was severely rutted, so much so that I had to put the truck into four-wheel drive just to keep from getting stuck. The truck bounced in and out of ruts so hard that papers fell off the dashboard (my filing system), and I actually had a little trouble hanging on to the steering wheel.

At the end of the roller-coaster ride, the scene unfolded in the twilight. The corral was constructed of old barbed wire draped from rotting post to rotting post, like old Christmas decorations that had been left up too long. The manure was ankle-deep and the only working lights available were the ones on the front of my truck. In the middle of the mess was an aging horse trailer. It was so badly rusted that even in the beam from my headlights, its original color was unrecognizable. Its tires were so flat that they melded into the muck that

they sat on. I could just see the outline of three hairy, horned creatures slowly moving around the confines of the corral, one more
slowly than the others. When they walked in front of the lights, I
could observe them in more detail. They all had the same brownish
black hair covering their torsos and their legs, all the way down to
their back hooves. They were not large creatures. About one-third the
size of a domestic cow, they each weighed approximately four hundred pounds, but for their size, they displayed very impressive horns.
In fact, from my angle, horns seemed to make up a large percentage
of their body mass. Their weaponry came out from the top of their
heads horizontally about six inches on each side, then shot straight up
at least a foot and a half. Each horn culminated in an extremely sharp
point, as if the creatures had some special yak horn–sharpening device that they used when no humans were looking. They turned to
glare at me in the headlights, insinuating that they were a united front
and I would be a fool to even get out of the truck.

The largest one, who also possessed the most impressive head-
gear, seemed to be breathing a little harder than the others and had
some discharge from both of his nostrils. Inevitably, he would have
to be the patient.

We have all seen television travel shows in which well-trained
yaks in Tibet are used to pack huge loads of supplies through the
Himalayas. Yet I didn't feel that these three in front of me had ever
packed gear to a Mount Everest base camp or even been handled at
all. It would turn out that my fears were not unfounded.

A knock on my window brought me back from my Travel Chan-
nel images. "Hey, Doc, thanks a lot for coming. You were the only
vet we could convince to try," Mr. Tyler reminded me as I stepped
out of the truck, which made me feel very special. Mr. Tyler was a tall,
thin man with a straggly beard and well-worn clothes. Mrs. Tyler was

a few steps behind him. She had a rather sad look to her. Her long blond hair hadn't seen a comb in a couple days and she was a little bent over from life's burdens. She had a general unhealthy, weak appearance, as if she would break if she even tripped over a rock. We reached the corral fence and stepped over its rusty remnants. A gate would have been way too much to ask.

Once we were in with the beasts, they began to realize that we weren't there just to admire their beauty. They moved out of the beam cast by the headlights into a darker, more discreet corner. We stood there, hoping they would reemerge. Mr. Tyler spoke up. "It's Jack, the big one, who's not feeling so good. I think we can run him into the trailer and treat him in there." Oh great, I thought. The chances of this working out were extremely low. And which one of the Tylers had come up with Jack the yak? In the dim light, Mr. Tyler and I picked up a couple of Aspen branches to drive them with and headed into the dark. The plan was to move the yaks back toward the trailer, then somehow into it. Mrs. Tyler got some grain from a metal trash can just outside the corral and put it inside the trailer to entice the animals. She would help guide them into the trailer once they got near it. We found the horned shadows in the far corner of the corral. Mr. Tyler and I got behind them and moved them toward the rear of the trailer, where Mrs. Tyler waited. As we got them closer to the trailer, they realized what the plan was and began to pick up speed. Right before they reached the entrance to our trap, Mrs. Tyler came out of the shadows, attempting to guide them into the open trailer door, but these yaks weren't buying. "Come on, get in there, you little buggers!" yelled Mr. Tyler. They completely ignored him and bolted in three different directions. Jack was moving incredibly well for an animal with a respiratory infection. He even managed to hold his head high and snorted in triumph after escaping our trap. Mr. Tyler swore and shook his fist at the elusive yaks. "We'll get you this time," he told them. Mrs. Tyler smiled, the first sign of emotion she had shown. She had obviously been in similar situations with her husband before and had a good idea how this was going to go. It would have been a good time to come up with a new plan, but there was no other plan. The trailer was our only option for capturing our patient, so we began to circle around again, and again they bolted. After the seventh try, they were beginning to slow down. On try number eleven, we seemed to be gaining, but we felt a little like the Three Stooges. "This is the last time you get away with it," Mr. Tyler managed to say between gasps for breath. Mrs. Tyler was now quietly laughing behind him.

All this movement and stress was causing everything the yaks had eaten in the last forty-eight hours to move on through. The corral floor was getting steadily more slippery and harder to maneuver. It was a bit like trying to run on an ice hockey rink covered with Jell-O.

On try number twelve, they gave up at the entrance to the trailer and reluctantly jumped in. Jack was the last one to make the leap, and in what I still claim was a final act of defiance, he shot out all that was left in his bowels. At the same time, I stepped up to close the door behind him. My feet slid out from under me and I landed square on my butt. The Tylers got a good laugh out of that. "I knew one of us was going to bite it eventually. Glad it wasn't me!" Mr. Tyler taunted. I got up, trying to act unaffected, and closed the door while the yaks munched on their grain.

I returned to the truck to gather my stethoscope, thermometer, and injectable antibiotics. Mrs. Tyler opened the door of the trailer to let her husband and me enter, then held the door closed behind us. We sorted out Jack, and then Mrs. Tyler let the other two out the back and slammed the door closed again. Now our patient could not escape. Mr. Tyler got a small rope around the ailing yak's horns and tied it off to the side of the trailer. Almost an hour after my arrival, I was ready to examine him. His temperature was a surprising 105 degrees and his lungs sounded congested. It was a good thing we had been persistent. The animal needed treatment and might not have made it without care. I pulled up a syringeful of long-acting antibiotic and dug through the thick hair to find some skin. The animal objected to the shot, taking a swat at me with a rear leg and shaking his horns in protest. This caused Mr. Tyler to snicker at me again. "Jack almost got you, Doc." He seemed to have forgotten how much he appreciated the fact I had come out; instead, I had become his evening entertainment. "Are we done?" he asked with a smile. I nodded and he slipped the rope off the animal's horns. "Open the door, honey!" he bellowed at Mrs. Tyler. But she already had opened it and was standing in the middle of the exit, watching the procedure. The newly released patient miraculously regained all of his strength, stampeding for his freedom. There was no doubt what was about to happen, and I figured my insurance company would have to be called about liability coverage. Jack exploded from the old trailer and the osteoporotic Mrs. Tyler disappeared. She had been hit head-on and knocked flat on her back. Mr. Tyler and I ran to her assistance. We found her in amazingly good shape. All her limbs seemed to be functional and she didn't have any neck pain. Maybe I won't have to call the insurance company tonight after all, I thought. We helped her to her feet and she brushed herself off. She appeared unscathed, but I would be checking with her over the next couple of weeks to be sure nothing cropped up. The yak's horns had not made contact. The animal's neck and chest must have knocked her over as he leaped out the back.

We walked her back toward the truck and I asked her again if she was all right. She smiled at me as if she could read my mind. "I'm fine; you don't have to worry." That gave me some relief and I scooted up onto the truck seat. The Tylers looked at me, awaiting some further instructions for the treatment of their yak. I wanted to hand Mr. Tyler a large syringe of antibiotic, tell him to give it to Jack in three days, and then speed off into the night. But I could not do this to Mrs. Tyler or Jack. Instead, I handed them some powdered antibiotic to mix with the feed three days hence, when the long-acting injection would have begun to wear off. They thanked me and I headed back up the obstacle course of a driveway.

I was exhausted. I decided to stop at a gas station for a candy bar and something to drink. I found my sugar fix and I walked up to the counter to pay. By now, it was almost 10:30 P.M., and the clerk looked at me skeptically over her glasses. "What are you doing out this late? Someone's kitty get sick?" she asked. "Well, not exactly," I responded. "Trust me, you don't want to know." "Well, whatever it was, looks like it worked you over pretty good" she said with a laugh, and stuck out her hand. "That'll be two dollars and fifty-six cents." I reached into my back pocket to grab my billfold and was very disappointed. My entire backside was caked with a present from Jack and my pocket was full of it. My billfold was covered and now so was my hand. I looked at the bewildered clerk, who was waiting patiently, and all I could think to say was, "Would you take a check?"

Intestinal Fortitude

I am often asked if animal injuries gross me out or make me sick. Many people tell me they could not handle the blood and don't know how I can deal with it on a regular basis. I'm sure most veterinarians don't think about wounds and injuries in that way. Caring for an animal is a given, but making it better as quickly as possible is our responsibility. We are trained to evaluate patients immediately, then come up with a plan to restore them to health. This training helps us focus in a way that keeps us from freaking out.

I remember dreading the first day of anatomy lab in veterinary school, wondering if I could handle it and being afraid of vomiting in front of my fellow students. I hung tough, but not all my classmates were as fortunate. As with many things in life, the first day was hard, but every day that followed got a little easier. We knew we had to get through these classes in order to be able to care for sick and injured animals once we were in practice. The problem is that as practicing veterinarians, we sometimes forget our clients have not had the same experiences and may not always react well to their own pets' injuries.

As a new graduate, I was often so involved in treating a wound that I would forget about what the owner was going through. Sometimes I would get so excited about a particular type of case that had not crossed my exam table before but had been discussed at length in a sleepy postlunch lecture a couple of years earlier that I would be oblivious to the owner's concern for his pet. I'm sure my excitement often made matters worse for a few of my early clients.

As time progressed, I began to gain enough confidence to work on a pet while explaining the procedure and prognosis to the owner at the same time. Still, it became apparent that some owners were not handling the sight of the wounds well, even getting a little woozy, despite my clinical explanations. For some reason, removing damaged tissue and suturing lacerations seemed to bother people as much as anything, and on one Colorado summer day, I would experience just how much.

I had been in the clinic most of the morning, neutering a couple of young cats the Humane Society had dropped off. They were not happy to be there, and it required a lot of patience to deal with them. Live-animal traps were the favorite feline transport device of the Humane Society, since many cats they brought in had had very little human exposure. Typically, such cats had been neglected or driven to the mountains and dropped off to fend for themselves. One could not blame them for their lack of trust, yet they still needed to be vaccinated and neutered.

The society volunteers would place a morsel of tuna in one end of the cage, and when the hungry kitty wandered in, they'd trip the release, causing the door to close behind the cat. While the caretakers had the best intentions, they were not willing to remove the cats from the traps—this honor was saved for the vet.

Since in the past both my employer and I had nearly been disfigured during the removal process, we'd had to devise a safe method to accomplish this. We would place a large plastic bag around the entire cage, connecting the open end to the gas anesthesia machine. After a few minutes, the feline would be sleeping soundly, keeping its stress, and ours, to a minimum. Although this proved to be a great way to handle feral cats, it was a time-consuming way to prepare an animal for surgery. So on the day in question, I was ready for some Rocky Mountain sunshine by the time I headed out to see an injured horse.

The animal belonged to Joe Taylor, a retired marine who now flew a Flight for Life chopper for a hospital in town. I always envied Joe a little because he was still in great shape at fifty-five. He maintained a regulation crew cut peppered with gray, and he treated his horse, Sarge, as if he was army issue. The big bay Morgan wanted for nothing. Joe spent at least one hour a day grooming him, and the lucky horse always received five-star hay. Joe was very proud of Sarge, and on the morning of the day I visited, he'd been horrified to find him with a four-inch cut on the end of his nose. The horse had come up against an exposed nail on the barn wall. I had no doubt that Joe would be sure to eliminate that problem the minute I had treated Sarge's injury.

The drive to the Taylor place was beyond picturesque. The road followed a small stream through a grassy valley that was guarded at the far end by a massive 13,000-foot peak. The scene always made me feel insignificant because I knew it had looked this way for thousands of years and would remain the same for thousands more. (That is, if it could escape the scourge of development ravaging the Rocky Mountains—but that's another story.)

On arrival, I pulled up to the neatly kept little barn and met Joe in the doorway. You could tell by his expression that he wished I could have gotten there earlier, but he was too nice a guy to mention that. "Good to see you, Doc," he said. Then, after the most minimal pause, he added, "Sarge doesn't look too good; he's right this way." He led me into the barn, where the big horse stood in cross ties. The four-inch cut ran from his right nostril to just above his lip on the left side. The edges were very smooth, as if the wound had been opened with a scalpel blade or, in Sarge's case, the point of a sixteen-penny nail.

Even though the blood had long since dried around the edges, I knew the scarring would be minimal. The face has such a concentrated blood supply that it heals beautifully and more quickly than other parts of the body, making the one who sews up a facial wound look like a hero.

After looking at the wound, I headed toward the truck to gather the needed supplies. "You won't need any painkillers or sedation for old Sarge—he's a tough one," Joe called after me. For a minute, I imagined the horse gritting his teeth as I forced the suture needle through the sensitive skin of his soft nose. Then I suggested that it would be easier for me if I used some sedation and local anesthetic. There was no way I would ever put an animal through unnecessary pain or anxiety when we had plenty of safe medications to prevent it.

I drew up a syringeful of tranquilizer and injected it into the Morgan's left jugular vein. As I returned to the truck for some lidocaine and instruments, Sarge started to get sleepy. His head dropped below his withers as he concentrated to keep his balance. Joe held his head steady, allowing me to inject the local anesthetic just under the skin along the edges of the wound. The tissue bubbled up where the numbing fluid was forced in, desensitizing the area I would be reconstructing. The whole time, Joe reassured the tranquilized horse that everything would be fine and that the scar would give him character. I think that I even caught Joe kissing Sarge's fuzzy brown ear when I was not supposed to be looking.

Next, I cleaned the wound aggressively with Betadine soap and positioned myself to repair it. The last stage before suturing is the removal of a tiny strip of tissue from the exposed edges in order to increase the probability of the skin pulling together as the wound heals. This procedure allows fresh blood to flow back into the wound. I could have sworn Joe choked a little as I did this. After clamping the needle in the appropriate instrument, I began the familiar pattern of suturing that would return the animal's nose to normal. By this time, I could feel Joe's warm breath on my neck. He had repositioned himself behind me and was looking over my shoulder in a sort of supervisory position. He spoke about how many times he had seen people with wounds ten times as severe and chuckled about colleagues who had not been able to handle such a gruesome sight.

I was not able to concentrate both on his conversation and the facial repair at the same time, so my brain automatically shut Joe off. After about ten minutes of sewing, I was carefully placing the last suture and explaining the after-care instructions to Joe. Sarge's nose looked a little Frankenstein-like with the ligatures in it, but he would be as good as new once they were removed. "Well, Joe," I said while observing my handiwork, "do you want to remove the sutures yourself, or do you want me to come back in a couple weeks and do it?" There was no response from behind me. I started to wonder if he thought my work was subpar or if he was just in awe.

I tried again, rubbing Sarge gently on the forehead to soothe him as I spoke. "So, Joe, what do you think?" Still no answer. I was beginning to think he was being just downright rude. I figured even if he was dissatisfied, he could at least come up with some type of polite answer. Straightening up slowly, I turned to face my client, but he wasn't there. Instead of admiring my work, he was flat on his back in the middle of the barn floor. He had passed out cold halfway through the repair, and I hadn't even noticed. After elevating his head and feet, I watched the color flow back into his face, and he slowly started to stir. Eventually, he regained consciousness and immediately began to apologize, visibly embarrassed. Even though Joe had experienced the sight of many grotesque human injuries during his life, the blood of an animal he so adored finished him.

Since that day, I have had many clients pass out while I was doing a procedure. I have lost them at their barns and in the clinic. Sometimes I've been able to catch them by reaching across the exam table before they met the floor, but more than once an owner's head has dented the drywall during a procedure to treat a loved pet. After the first few times this happened, I got better at recognizing the warning signs, including the lack of conversation, pale face, and glazed-over eyes. But I've learned that probably the best clue to a potential fainter is if the person brags about not being queasy.

Biker Dog

The Rocky Mountain region is full of fascinating people from all walks of life, and one day I found myself face-to-face with one of the more interesting ones. Mama, as she was known around town, was clutching her beloved dog while I cleaned up the "road rash" on his left hip.

The first time I had observed Mama, I was having dinner with some friends at a local Italian restaurant. We were in the middle of eating some form of pasta in a marinara sauce when I noticed the noise level in the room was on the increase in order to compete with the incessant barking coming from the parking lot. It was a crystal-clear mountain evening, so all the windows and doors were wide open for the comfort of the patrons. Unfortunately, this allowed the ear-piercing yipping to flow through the restaurant unchallenged. About the time that I thought the conversation could not get any louder, a stout woman at the bar with a black Harley leather jacket, a long gray braid, and arms completely covered by tattoos turned from her beer to the row of motorcycles parked out front. She proceeded to scream at the top of her lungs, "Megadeth! Megadeth! Shut yer pie hole!" This announcement quieted the entire restaurant—but not the barking dog outside. It took a few more reprimands for Megadeth to back down and the restaurant to return to a more natural conversation level.

I was dying to get a peek at the demon outside, so I faked a trip to the rest room in order to peer out into the parking lot. I was more than surprised to see that the only canine on the premises was a tiny Chihuahua seated squarely on the seat of a motorcycle, staring longingly into the bar. He was sporting a black leather vest that was edged with rhinestones and had a skull and crossbones on the back. The attire and motorcycle seemed to give the small dog the confidence of a German shepherd, yet he looked more like some kind of postnuke mutant.

His eyes bulged from their sockets, and his larger-than-life paper-thin ears added to his alien appearance. Mama had squelched his confidence for the moment, so he eventually crawled into one of the saddlebags that hung off each side of the Harley. In fact, I learned later, this is the position that Megadeth was most commonly seen in. He would sit in the saddlebag, his head sticking out the top just enough for his ears to catch the breeze. His eyes were protected by a pair of black "doggles," which matched the goggles that Mama wore. The two were a common sight in our mountain area, cruising to-gether up and down the winding roads. But on this day, they were in the clinic, and the road trips were going to have to be postponed for a while.

Mama explained that Megadeth had been nestled in his usual position when she swerved to miss a large rock that had fallen onto the pavement, as rocks often do when the ice melts in the spring. She had been able to avoid the rock, but Megadeth was ejected from his leather sidecar onto the concrete, where he slid on his side for about ten feet. The fall and subsequent slide had sheared off the hair and some skin from the little dog's side.

Mama had flown up our driveway like Evel Knievel and burst into the clinic with the little dog cradled in her muscular arms. He was wrapped in her black leather jacket, which was soaked through with Chihuahua blood. She gently laid him on the exam table and her tears began to flow. This wasn't unusual, of course. Often when people bring an injured pet to the veterinarian, they feel that they have com-

pleted their task of being in charge and can turn over the reins of
control to the veterinarian. Then the true emotions come through.
The tough lady was now looking at me more like a frightened child
than a seasoned biker.

After giving the little guy a thorough exam, I realized that the
only serious injury he had sustained was a potato chip–size open sore
over the hip. The skin from this section had been left behind on the
pavement, and what remained looked like raw meat sprinkled with
tiny pebbles ground in from the slide. I explained to Mama that he
was going to be fine but that the wound would require a lot of care
over the next month. Since there was really nothing left to suture, it
would have to remain open and heal in from the edges. Mama
agreed to care for Megadeth's injuries diligently, so we got started
right away.

Hands that could bend steel gently held the trembling pup while
I picked the rocks out of the dried blood that coated the lesion. Like
most owners, she was a little nervous about holding her injured pet
while treatment was being performed. As Megadeth struggled to
avoid my cleansing, Mama's grip tightened around his neck. I asked
her to ease off a couple of times, but as soon as he flinched, her
adrenaline kicked in and the strong hands contracted back to full
force. Unfortunately, too much restraint around the neck of a small
breed with bulging eyes, such as shih tzus, Boston terriers, and this
Chihuahua, can dramatically increase the pressure in the animal's
head. Megadeth's patience had just about run out, so he made a final
attempt to turn his head and bite my hand. Mama panicked even
more, her grip tightened further, and the dog's right eye popped
completely out of its socket! It hung there, dangling only by the tiny
eye muscles and optic nerve. Hollywood special-effects people could
not have produced a more horrifying scene.

When Mama saw the expelled eyeball, she began to gag and ran from the room in tears. I yelled for Christie and she came running in to help. We quickly anesthetized the little canine, and after a couple minutes of manipulation, we had the elusive eyeball back in its socket. I had been through this many times with small exophthalmic dogs that had ended up on the losing end of a canine dispute and had been brought in with displaced peepers, but never had I seen it happen right in front of me.

In order to keep the eyeball in place, the lids had to be sutured closed until the inflammation receded, allowing the eye to achieve its original fit. Taking advantage of the anesthetic, we also finished cleaning the wound on the dog's hip.

I went out to the waiting room to talk with Mama while Christie waited for the patient to wake up. After I explained to Mama that her beloved pet would be fine and probably retain most of the sight in the newly reset eye, her fear turned to guilt. She felt terrible about her excessive use of force but seemed to feel better when I exaggerated just a little about how commonly this exact situation occurred.

We loaded her up with anti-inflammatories and antibiotics and sent the pair on their way. This time, the motorcycle pulled out of the driveway at a much slower pace.

I wondered several times over the next week how Mama and Megadeth were getting along. The answer came to me as I was driving down the highway to check on a lame horse and saw a woman on a motorcycle pass me on a double yellow line. Yes, it was Mama, with Megadeth in his usual spot. He sat in his tough-guy stance, except a couple of new accessories had been added. On top of his head was a helmet fashioned out of half a black plastic ball. An old shoestring wrapped under his jaw held it on, and over his right eye was a tiny leather patch that would have made even the fiercest of pirates proud.

Even after the eye was completely healed and the sutures had been removed, I would occasionally spot him sporting the patch like a badge of honor. Mama said it made him feel more like a "real tough biker dog." Eventually, she forgot which eye she had made the patch for. Thus, in the months that followed, he could be seen with it over either eye, but the effect was the same—for Megadeth and for onlookers.

A Hog in the House

Pets obviously come in every size, shape, and color. They can be mammalian, reptilian, or avian. Pigs are probably one of the more unusual pets, especially when they live in the house. Being from rural Iowa—that is, hog country—I have to admit that I found it a little strange when Korean potbellied pigs became so popular as house pets. The fad seemed to sweep the country, and these funny animals became quite an expensive commodity. It became almost a status symbol to own one. Potbellied pigs are relatively small hogs as long as they are not overfed. But since restricting feed is nearly impossible for most pet lovers, including me, the result can be a two-hundred-plus-pound porcine pal sharing the couch. They are meant to live on a diet of fruits and vegetables, yet I have observed these spoiled potbellies ingesting everything from marshmallows to cornflakes.

Their skin is dark and almost scaly, with sparse long hairs protruding like porcupine quills. Since they are not big on looks, the name "potbellied" is well deserved. Their pendulous abdomens hang so low to the ground, they often drag on the floor as the animals wander about the house.

Loading these misshapen porcine companions in the car can be a little tough, so we usually have to see them on their own turf. Most commonly, they are sprawled out on the kitchen floor, a cushy dog bed between their tough hide and the linoleum. Mrs. Chandler's pig, Bacon, was no exception. He lay snoring in his place of honor near the heat vent when I arrived in response to his owner's call. Mrs. Chandler had to step over his 150-pound body to get to the refrigerator, the stove, and the counter, where the children sat eating breakfast. She moved about the room gracefully, stepping over the pig without missing a beat, as if he were one of the kitchen furnishings. After all, this was where he spent most of his time, and the Chandlers had accepted that. I had witnessed this routine several times before due to the fact that Bacon required a hoof trim and vaccinations once a year.

The Chandlers had a beautiful modern kitchen with dark granite countertops and stainless-steel appliances, but a couple of features were clearly not standard Home Depot issue: The refrigerator and oven had large metal latches screwed onto the doors. When my curiosity got the best of me on a previous visit and I asked about these, the family informed me that Bacon was capable of opening the doors and stealing the contents inside, so they had installed these burglar-proof latches.

I arrived that day to take care of Bacon's annual treatment. Some might think this would be a fairly easy task, but these would be people who have had very little experience with pigs. Bacon always had to be anesthetized for his pedicure. He hated the injection and screamed at the top of his lungs in anticipation. The same scene played out every time. Bacon ran around the kitchen squealing and skating on the slick floor as I chased after him with the syringe clutched in my hand like a knife. I had tried sneaking up on him, even crawling across the floor on my hands and knees, but he always spotted me at the last minute. Finally, I would corner him long enough to inject the drugs, and Bacon would drift off, at last ending the ear-piercing part of the ordeal. By the time the excessive hoof was cut off and the appropriate vaccinations given, he would already have begun to come around, and he would be fully recovered in time for his next meal. This day played out no differently, and within an hour I was on my way to the next case, after the usual thanks and apologies from Mrs. Chandler for my inconvenience.

About two weeks after my trip to see Bacon, Mrs. Chandler called me out again to see not only the pampered pig but also his best friend, Buck, a yellow Labrador. The problem was that they had both escaped through the Invisible Fence and proceeded to eat an entire bag of cat food that was stored in the garage. Because the cat food was much higher in protein than they were used to, a constant stream of pungent diarrhea was coming from both animals. Much to Mrs. Chandler's disappointment, Bacon had made it back to his favorite spot in the kitchen before it hit him, turning the room into a barn lot in a matter of minutes.

If that wasn't bad enough, he dribbled through almost every room in the house before Mrs. Chandler could run him back into the yard. By this time, her normally perfectly styled hair was no longer perfect, and perspiration had caused her makeup to run. She was practically crying in frustration as she mumbled something about the Invisible Fence.

When I cornered Bacon in the yard to treat him with some bismuth solution for his overactive bowels, I noticed the large collar around his thick neck, hidden under his fourth double chin. There I found the typical plastic box with two metal prongs to transfer a minimal current to the animal if it crossed the underground electric barrier. I have to admit that I'd never found one of these contraptions on a pig before. Bacon's collar had had to be extended with an extra nylon strap, since it had been designed to fit a dog's neck. Buck also was sporting his "escapeproof" collar, which brought up the question of how both animals had been able to leave the electrified backyard and get to the cat food in the garage.

Mrs. Chandler saw the bewilderment on my face and began to explain before I could even ask. "Let me show you what's going on here," she said. "Bacon is a little more than your average pet." She left Buck and Bacon in the backyard with their collars in place. Making sure that the Invisible Fence was activated, she placed a bowl of table scraps just out of reach across the invisible barrier.

Then I followed her into the house, where we watched the scene unfold through a kitchen window. At first, Bacon and Buck circled in the yard, acting casual, trying to ignore the bait. But once Bacon decided that his owner and I were not coming back outside, he pointed his snout at the bowl with a look of determination, at which point he transformed into a wild boar ready to attack his prey in the bush. Next, his wrinkled body began to twitch and shake as if he was starting to have a seizure. A crescendoing squeal came from his open mouth, and his poor excuse for a tail spun like a helicopter blade. Buck was going through a similar procedure just a couple of steps behind the pig. Then Bacon's eyes closed tightly and he lunged across the underground wire, with Buck on his heals. Bacon had figured out how to psych himself up to run past the shock of the fence, and he had taught Buck to do the same.

After the two were happily munching on their prize, Mrs. Chandler turned to me. "I guess pigs are just too darn smart for these gadgets," she said. "I just don't know how I'm going to keep him in, and now he's taught my dog how to escape also." From my rural upbringing, I knew that swine could be all but impossible to contain. They use their tough shovel-like noses to root under fences and easily exit their pens, always certain something is more interesting and potentially tasty in the world outside. In farm country, pigs are perpetually destroying gardens and ruining neighborly relations.

Over the years, the Chandlers fortified their yard countless times, but Bacon always managed to escape, followed by any family pet that was up for a romp. After he had ingested all the contents of the neighborhood gardens, he would then raid the garbage cans. These little binges did not do anything for the Chandlers' popularity, but they didn't seem to be able to stop him. Finally, as Bacon began to age, he spent more time in the house and less time pillaging the countryside.

Eventually, he became such a sedentary old pig that the destruction completely came to an end—a relief for everyone involved, especially the Chandlers.

I hadn't heard much about Bacon for several months, but then we received a call one morning from Mrs. Chandler, who wanted me to stop by and check on him. He was lying in his old spot in the middle of the kitchen, sleeping off breakfast, when I walked in. "He's not moving around much anymore, but his appetite is still good," she told me. "I pretty much give him whatever he wants these days." Beside him was a dog bowl full of apples and chocolate-chip cookies. It was hard to feel too sorry for Bacon.

I examined him, only to find some arthritic joints, typical of a pig old enough for a senior citizen discount. "He's just getting older," I explained to Mrs. Chandler, and suggested she start him on some supplements for his joints. "I guess you're relieved he's not terrorizing the neighborhood anymore," I added as I patted his engorged stomach. "I guess he'll be your last pet pig?"

No response came from Mrs. Chandler. I looked up to see her rather befuddled expression. "Well, actually, we thought some young blood might keep Bacon a little more active." She walked to the back door and pushed it open just a crack. A tiny potbellied piglet tore into the room, made a couple of laps around it, and slid to a stop in front of me. His eyes twinkled and his snout was already covered with dirt from the backyard. "Meet Pork Chop," Mrs. Chandler said. "I just couldn't resist him."

Foster Family

Everyone has heard the old adage that people tend to look like their pets, and I've found that it is often true. Most veterinarians will tell you that animals and their owners often have the same medical problems, as well. Whether it is obesity or hyperthyroidism, the number of times they have the same affliction is almost uncanny. The tough part about this correlation is informing an owner of his pet's situation. Often the person may have been dealing with the condition himself for years, so he knows what his pet will have to go through. For obvious reasons, telling someone that her cat is overweight, for example, can be a little uncomfortable for everyone involved and certainly disappointing for the cat. "Light" feline food often has a consistency similar to sawdust, even though it is just what the overindulgent cat needs. Another hard one is telling a senior citizen that her sixteen-year-old poodle is suffering from old age and explaining the curses of that condition. She will give me a knowing nod, indicating that she can relate, but under the surface lies the acknowledgment of her own mortality.

Thomas Gertsen had been a client for many years but had never disclosed any information about his own ailments. He was a very conscientious pet owner, sparing no expense when it came to his beloved cat, Andre. Thomas was a short, heavyset man who was beginning to gray a little around the temples. He was a confirmed bachelor and spent his days fixing people's computer problems. Andre, coincidentally, looked very similar. He was a stocky little yellow tabby who was beginning to gray around the muzzle.

Andre usually came in only for his annual vaccinations and teeth cleaning, but one day Thomas brought him in because of some abnormal behavior. The cat had begun to drink more water and urinate more often than normal, both signs of an internal problem. After I found a high level of sugar in Andre's urine and blood, my suspicions were confirmed: He had diabetes and would require daily insulin injections to treat it.

A large percentage of pet owners would not be able to handle this commitment, but after an explanation of the treatment he would be required to perform, Thomas nodded and accepted the responsibility with enthusiasm. Then he reached into his pocket and produced a glucometer, along with a couple of insulin syringes. "I have been a diabetic for twenty years, so having two of us in the house won't be much of a hardship!" he declared. I had no argument with that and proceeded to show him how to give Andre the shots.

Thomas brought his pet in every month after that so we could test the blood-sugar level, adjusting the insulin levels accordingly. Since Thomas was very diligent and Andre quite accommodating, it was relatively easy to regulate the medication. For two years, the routine continued, and so did Andre's stable health. But one day I received a call from Thomas, who said that our patient had lost some weight and was drinking and urinating abnormally again, not really the kind of information I wanted to hear.

When he arrived in the exam room, the cat was severely dehydrated and lethargic. His beautiful yellow hair had lost its elasticity, and Andre's breath smelled a little like acetone. Unfortunately, I knew what the diagnosis would be, but I had to back it up with blood work. Thomas knew also; he had been involved in long conversations with his own physician about the potential effects of long-term diabetes. We placed a catheter in Andre's right cephalic vein and started some IV fluids to combat his dehydration. After making Andre comfortable in a kennel, Thomas went home to wait for the lab results. Within a few hours, we had them, confirming our worst fears. Andre was suffering from kidney failure—not just a mild case but a complete shutdown. The poor cat had not produced any urine in the last three hours, even after half a liter of fluids. Thomas stroked Andre's dull coat as I explained the situation. He fought back the tears, but a few managed to escape down his pale cheeks. He nodded knowingly as I told him we needed to put his friend out of his misery.

Telling him to take all the time he needed, I left them alone together in the exam room to say their good-byes. I always feel somewhat helpless in these situations, knowing that not even the most well-chosen words can make things less painful. As veterinarians, we just do the best we can to be there for both human and animal. In about five minutes, Thomas opened the door, indicating that he was as ready as he was going to be. He wanted to stay with Andre, so Christie came in to hold the cat while I injected the euthanasia solution into the catheter that we had placed earlier. Andre drifted off quietly as the rest of us stared down at him silently. Finally, Thomas eked out a "Thank you," but Christie and I could only nod in acknowledgment; we both knew that if we spoke, we would not be able to maintain our composure.

Euthanasia is the hardest aspect of veterinary practice, yet it is one of the most important. Many preveterinary students have put an end to their career aspirations after assisting with this procedure. Some might think that it would get easier with time, but they would be very wrong.

It was hard to see Thomas leave the clinic in tears and alone. He placed the empty cat carrier into the backseat of his Honda Civic and pulled away. The rest of that day, none of us was too cheery. The loss of Andre had left us all a little depressed, and we could visualize Thomas sitting alone in his house that evening.

It was almost closing time and getting dark when my boss phoned in after finishing a horse call. He had found two tiny kittens at the intersection of two gravel roads on his way home. The fate of their mother was unknown, but they were hungry and cold. He had scooped them up and was bringing them into the clinic for the night. "I think we'll need some help with these two," my boss said as he carried in the kittens. "What do you suppose Thomas Gertsen is up to tonight?"

Agreeing that we would be too busy to care for the kittens, I looked up Thomas's number and dialed. The phone rang several times before a quiet voice came through on the other end. "Thomas, hey, this is Jeff, from the veterinary clinic," I said. "I'm especially sorry to bother you now, but I have a little bit of a problem and am hoping you can help me out. We have found some abandoned kittens that will require regular bottle-feeding during the night, and we're just too overwhelmed to do it."

There was a long pause on the other end. Then he said, "This really isn't a good time. I'm so upset about my loss . . . but Andre would have wanted me to help them. If it's only for tonight, I'll do my part."

"I'll drop them off, then," I responded. "Thank you so much for your help."

Gathering up an armload of kitten milk replacer, I headed for his house. Thomas had a modest single-story home in a mountain subdivision. The place was a little depressing that night. Only the living room light was on, and I saw Thomas pop up from his chair to greet us. I met him at the door with the kittens, which were in a small cardboard box with a bath towel for padding. His eyes were red from crying, and he stared downward to hide them from me.

I shoved the box into his arms, trying to act rushed. He fought back a small smile upon looking into the container, but he couldn't cover up the little bit of happiness that crept into his eyes. "Thanks again, Thomas. Could you drop them off at the clinic in the morning?" I asked as I set the cans of milk down on the cement step. He nodded in affirmation, and I hurried off. As I left, I noticed he turned on a few more lights in the house.

The next morning, Thomas did not show up with the kittens. He called in about 11:30 to say that one of the little guys had not eaten very much during the night but that he would work with the kitten for the rest of the day. He said he would definitely drop them off the next morning, however. But the next day came and went with no sign of Thomas or the kittens. Finally, on the third day, Thomas called the clinic and wanted to talk to me. "I'm afraid these kittens don't want to leave," he explained. "I've tried to take them back, but they don't want to go. I guess I'll just have to keep them, if it's okay."

I told him that we'd talk it over but that I thought it would be okay. I hung up the phone and my boss asked me, "So, what's the deal?"

"They'll be in for vaccinations in a few weeks," I replied. "Mission accomplished."

Fish Out of Water

Dating can be a little difficult for a young veterinarian who's single. Rural areas tend not to have large populations of available young women. The combination of few potential prospects, long workdays, and after-hours emergencies left much to be desired with regard to my social life. Rural Colorado was a far cry from nightlife in the city, where there were clubs and happy hours. Friends always had that "really nice girl" they wanted to set me up with, but such women usually made for an interesting first and only date. Sometimes clients would have single daughters, but when they realized that I lived in a rented cabin and drove a practically antique Jeep, their enthusiasm waned. Just because I had "Dr." in front of my name didn't mean I produced the kind of income that physicians with a human clientele did. Just when I was about to give up, new staff members started showing up at one of the guest ranches served by the practice.

This meant a lot of young women from all over the country would be moving to the area for temporary jobs, as they did every year. The summer help spent three to four months doing everything from cleaning toilets to taking guests out on trail rides. Most years, I didn't get to know the staff that well, but one particular summer the entire herd of horses at one guest ranch contracted a respiratory disease known as strangles, so my services were needed two to three times a week as the disease spread rapidly through the herd.

This bacterial ailment is typically carried in by a new horse and spreads like wildfire from there. This incredibly contagious affliction is called strangles because it most commonly affects the lymph nodes around the lower neck, causing them to fill with pus and press against the windpipe. It is typical to see strangles horses standing around the corral with their necks extended, trying to get air. Fortunately, most of these animals are fairly easy to treat, but the cure is not for the weak-stomached. The pus-filled lymph nodes must be drained, allowing the copious amounts of stinky white fluid to escape. Antibiotics are often used in severe cases.

Due to the frequency of my visits to the ranch that summer, I got to know the staff a little better than usual, especially one of the wranglers. Marion was a beautiful blonde with big brown eyes and a warm smile. She had extremely short hair, which I didn't think much about at the time, but after a little reconnaissance, I found out that she had survived cancer and a liver transplant during the past year. She was only twenty-one at the time. After this life-changing experience, Marion turned down a banking job in New York and headed for Colorado. She wanted to do something totally different to help with her recovery—which proved fortunate for me, as it turned out.

We became friends as the summer progressed, and she decided to stay on into the fall, long after the rest of the staff would have returned to college. She had already graduated, so I had time to develop a game plan without appearing overly interested. The truth is, it got to the point where I was making up reasons to show up at the ranch and see Marion. But I had to walk a fine line so that no one would catch on. One advantage of being a single male who's over thirty is learned patience when it comes to dating.

My opportunity eventually came when an overly aggressive suitor showed up to take Marion out one fall evening. I happened to be at the ranch, and Marion wanted me to act as if she and I already had plans. I played it casual. "Well, I guess if it will help you out . . . I could take you to dinner." This nonchalant attitude could have backfired, I realize now, but in this case, it worked as planned. Within a few weeks, we were dating, but her time at the ranch was quickly running out as the tourist season came to an end. She headed home over the holidays for a month, during which I missed her every second. In January, she was back in Colorado, and before we knew it, we were an item.

Usually, I'd reach a point in the dating process (which I had begun to call anything that lasted past a date or two) when I would begin looking for things not to like in a current girlfriend. But this time, there seemed to be nothing to dislike, and this was making me more than just a little nervous. Marion was obviously a very special person to have lived through what she had, and she had a great attitude about life. We also had very similar interests, including a mutual love of animals—an important attribute if you're going to spend a lot of time with a veterinarian.

In most relationships, there comes a time when it is appropriate to meet the significant other's family and friends. The wedding of an old friend of Marion's back in Connecticut provided the opportunity in our case.

Marion was originally from southern Connecticut, so the first part of our trip was devoted to meeting parents and extended family. When that stress was over, I was able to relax enough to notice that this was the land of Martha Stewart. Beautiful old Colonial homes, immaculately groomed grounds, and quaint main streets were magically protected from strip malls and big-box stores. SUVs equipped with golden retrievers and driven by beautiful women with perfect bobbed hairdos dotted the roads. This was a long way from the small Iowa farming community where I'd grown up, but fortunately Marion had bought me some new clothes for the trip and decked me out in the uniform of the Northeast: a blue blazer and khakis. I was glad of it, because I realized immediately that my usual dog hair–covered flannel shirts and dirty jeans were not going to cut it here.

Even after surveying the surroundings and realizing, as they say, that we weren't in Kansas anymore, I still was not prepared for the sort of wedding we attended. The bride's father was the CEO of an international corporation, and the wedding took place at just one of the homes in their collection. It was a huge white Colonial with black shutters and a circular driveway. Hundreds of flowers had been strategically placed throughout the yard just for this special day, but they gave the impression that they had grown there of their own accord. A fresh slate walkway led to the backyard, where the festivities were already beginning under a huge tent strung with tiny white lights. It was *Father of the Bride* gone wild. In each corner was a full bar, manned by three extremely attentive and well-groomed bartenders. Other staff bustled their way from chafing dish to chafing dish, preventing the horror of horrors—less-than-overflowing trays of pink tenderloin medallions. I sympathized with the staff, feeling a little more comfortable with them than with many of the guests.

The bulk of the temporary Taj Mahal contained round tables draped with crisp white tablecloths. Eight elaborate place settings adorned each table, with multiple forks surrounding every plate. For me, this meant embarrassing moments to come as I tried to guess which one was for what. Roses at the peak of bloom were stuffed so tightly in vases at the center of each table that I thought their containers might explode.

At one end of the tent stood a long table with even more extravagant flower arrangements, obviously set aside for the wedding party. At the opposite end, large black speakers were being set up for the night's entertainment. I began to feel more than a little out of place in this opulent setting. Midwestern wedding receptions were usually carried out in the basement of the church. For a small donation, a group of women in the church would make sandwiches, Jell-O salad, and punch for the guests, while the cake was often put together by a family member. Having grown up in a Methodist community, I was used to the strongest ingredient in the punch being cranberry juice, and dancing was not generally encouraged. But this was a different world, and I knew I would have to adjust—quickly. A good performance would not only impress Marion but would also increase my chances of gaining the acceptance of her friends, whom I had not met before that day. This was important, since every man knows that he doesn't stand a chance until all the girls his girlfriend has ever known have given the thumbs-up. So the pressure was on. This might be my only chance, I realized, and I didn't even have the home-court advantage.

One unfortunate aspect of my date being in the wedding party was that she would not be able to sit with me. Her place was with the rest of the bridesmaids at the head table. Normally, this would not have been a big deal, but I was so far out of my element that I dreaded a two-hour dinner without her. The guests began to filter into the tent and search out their place cards. Having scoped out my seat early on, I watched as my table filled up with smartly dressed urban couples. Drawing in a deep breath, I could not put off the inevitable any longer and headed for my assigned seat.

The faces around me went silent as I pulled my chair up to the table and fumbled with my napkin. I soon found out that they all knew one another and worked with the bride in New York. Why I was seated with this group of Manhattanites was a bit of a mystery, but since I knew no one except Marion, I supposed this table was as good as any. They observed me with great interest, asking the usual questions about career and where I lived. Eventually, they came to the conclusion that I was some combination of Grizzly Adams and James Herriot. They were at least clear about the fact that I was definitely not the typical Wall Street type they were accustomed to.

Finally, after an uncomfortable lull in the conversation and a lot of staring in my direction, one man spoke up, asking a question I could handle. He was a middle-aged fellow with one of those comb-overs that would not have done well in a stiff breeze. "I've got a bulldog that was in the kennel last week while we were in the Hamptons," he began, "and now he has a loud cough. In fact, it's keeping us awake at night. What do you think?" The whole group awaited my answer with great anticipation. Thank goodness it was a fairly easy absentee diagnosis, and I felt myself straightening up in the chair to explain it. "The pup obviously picked up kennel cough during his doggy hotel stint," I said. "It's the most common disease that dogs pass back and forth in tight quarters. A couple of weeks' worth of antibiotics and the pooch should be back to normal." The man seemed to be relieved by this information and settled back to enjoy his lobster bisque.

The rest of my tablemates then began to stir, as all of them had a few questions about their pets' illnesses. They took turns asking me for veterinary advice about everything from feline bladder infections to ear mites in dogs. Some practitioners might have been offended by being pressed for free advice, but I was elated to have the conversation turn to something I understood. The eccentricities of the stock market had always been a hard topic for me to grasp. Once everyone seemed happy with my responses to their inquiries, I was no longer an outsider. In fact, they completely accepted me for the rest of the evening. Our table was responsible for the loudest chatter and most laughter, giving me high boyfriend marks for the event. But I can't take full credit—the open bar may have contributed a little.

Somewhere between the filet mignon and the wedding cake, the band started up and the dancing commenced. The lead singer was good enough to have brought down the house in Vegas, and he was accompanied by backup vocalists and several instruments. The band's repertoire ranged from *Big Chill* tunes to the best of James Brown, the kind of songs that take you back to where you heard them the first time. It's amazing how music can bring back memories that include familiar sights, sounds, and smells. Observing the people dancing in the lighted tent, I was reminded how weddings can stir up the romantic in people.

Couples who had been married for decades were pulling each other close and exchanging kisses as if they were the only ones in the room. Single women started looking at their boyfriends, maybe wondering why they hadn't been asked yet, and people without escorts just tended to drink more as the evening progressed. When the band started in on their rendition of "Only Fools Fall in Love," I noticed a couple of young bachelors staring at my date, my cue to ask her to dance.

Weddings are contagious. A year later, Marion and I were walking down the aisle. Even now, after ten years of marriage, I still can't wait to get home at night to see her.

Overexposed

 More often than not, small dogs spend their lives thinking they are Great Danes or Saint Bernards. They act like big dogs in small-dog suits. Unfortunately, this way of thinking doesn't always pay off for them. One of these typical small dogs was a tough little Yorkshire terrier named David. He would come to see us once a year for an exam and vaccinations. David came in with his two biggest fans—his human, Miss Davis, and his protector, Goliath, a 120-pound German shepherd. Goliath's main job in life was to keep David from getting killed by other members of his own species.

Miss Davis, an attractive middle-aged woman, was just glad that we were there for her pets. She was one of those clients whom we were always glad to see come through the door because she was so happy and appreciative. According to Miss Davis, she had put dog fencing around her whole yard, but David had dug out a small tunnel so that he could come and go as he pleased. Every time she tried to plug the hole, the determined little David would just find a way to open it up again. The problem was that he loved to harass the neighbor's two full-grown malamutes. He would burrow through his escape hatch and taunt the big boys next door until they couldn't take it anymore. The trick was that once he had pushed them to the limit, David would scurry back into the safety of his own yard. He would then hide behind Goliath and yip at his frustrated pursuers through the fence. David knew they didn't have any interest in coming over the fence to take on his bodyguard.

The plan worked well until one snowy mountain day in March. David was going through his usual routine of antagonizing the neighbor dogs, but when he turned to make a run for home, he realized that snow had fallen off a nearby tree while he was gone and was now covering the entrance to his tunnel. He could not find it fast enough, and, sadly, Goliath could do nothing to help his little friend. The German shepherd barked and growled, tearing at the metal fence, but he couldn't stop the attack. Little David didn't stand a chance. The noise did bring Miss Davis bolting out of the house, and she was able to rip David from the jaws of death by beating off the attackers with a shovel.

Even a small amount of blood in fresh snow gives the appearance that a mass murder has been committed, so Miss Davis was in quite a panic when she called the clinic to tell us she was on the way in. Christie and I continued to see the patients that were in the waiting room, and about ten minutes later, Miss Davis threw open the door, holding the bloody little fuzz ball in her arms. She ran past the rest of the clients and into the exam room, her eyes red and puffy from crying. She placed him gently on the table, then looked to me. "Please help him, please," she said softly. "You've got to save him." I felt as bad for her as I did for the little terrier.

I started to examine the victim, looking for any major damage. The poor little guy was very scared and tried to escape the examination by climbing up his owner's chest. His little paws were scraping back and forth as fast as they could while Miss Davis leaned over the table, attempting to hold him down. Unfortunately, she had worn a low-cut, loose-fitting blouse without undergarments. In her haste to save David, she hadn't bothered to put on something more practical. She didn't realize that in David's panic, he was actually pulling down her blouse. The next thing I knew, I was standing across from a mostly topless woman, with only a bloody terrier between us.

My face was so red-hot, you could have fried an egg on it. I had no idea what to say or do, so I just kept working on David's wounds. I was trying hard to concentrate only on the little dog. At no point in veterinary school had this situation ever been discussed. I gave David some sedative, and he relaxed just enough for me to get him back to the treatment room. Miss Davis casually pulled herself back together and headed for the waiting room until we could give her more information on David's status. She was too worried about her pet to be embarrassed.

We shaved the hair away from the wounds and got David cleaned up enough to conclude that he was free of life-threatening lesions. He had lost some blood but not enough to warrant a transfusion.

After his wounds were all treated and the sedative wore off, David started to act like himself again almost immediately. In fact, he got a little cocky, growling at another dog in a treatment kennel nearby. I decided that it would be best to keep David overnight for observation, so we placed him in a kennel away from any other dogs to decrease the possibility of a repeat performance.

Back in the waiting room, Miss Davis waited for the report, but I wasn't looking forward to giving it to her, even though it was good news. Facing her wasn't going to be easy after her accidental exposure in the exam room. I finally walked out to meet her, quickly spewing out the details of David's condition. "He just has some minor flesh wounds. He'll be fine, just fine." I took a deep breath and waited nervously for her reaction.

Her face widened in a big smile. "Oh, thank you so much," she said. "I was afraid we were going to lose him. There was so much blood." She gave me a peck on the cheek and headed home—to put on more clothes, I guessed.

David went home the next day, and as she paid the bill, Miss Davis made a joke about how she wasn't really an exhibitionist. She and I have laughed about that day many times since, but there is still a little awkwardness when I see her in the checkout line at the local grocery.

Too Much Information

As I began to practice, I discovered that many responsibilities of the veterinary practitioner are not discussed in school. These responsibilities fall under the "Learn as you go" category, and the role of counselor/psychologist is one of the most prominent. New veterinarians would expect to need these skills for discussing such things as the loss of a pet or a tough treatment decision, yet it's the non-veterinary-related problems that people continue to surprise me with. Sometimes I wish that I had taken a few more psychology courses before graduation and studied a little less chemistry. The elements on the periodic table don't seem quite as relevant now, but these counseling situations come up almost daily in practice. A few of them stand out in my mind.

One of the most memorable involved a concerned father. I had treated all of the Stanleys' pets over the years, but one day I was at their ranch to take care of one of their horses, who was suffering from an upper respiratory infection. It was a beautiful fall day in the Rockies, and I was very glad to get out of the office to enjoy it. The aspens were just starting to turn their golden yellow, and the sky was more cobalt than blue. There was no place else I would rather have been that day—that is, until Mr. Stanley said, in his deep Barry White voice, "Doc, I need to talk to you about something when we finish." My heart sank, for I was sure he had a complaint about something the staff or I had done or said.

Mr. Stanley was a tall man in his mid-forties, with a long beard and unkempt long blond hair. A rather intimidating figure, he looked as if he should be getting off a Viking ship to conquer new lands, and now he wanted to discuss something with me. I racked my brain, trying to think of what it might be. None of his animals had died under our care; in fact, he always seemed happy with the treatment they received. I dragged out the horse's treatment as long as I could, but eventually I couldn't delay any longer. I put a label with instructions on a bottle of antibiotics and leaned up against the truck, prepared to defend myself. Crossing my arms and setting my jaw, I braced myself for the onslaught.

Mr. Stanley sat down on a stump, rubbing the head of his Irish wolfhound, from whose stomach I had surgically removed several rocks when he was just a puppy. Mr. Stanley lighted a Marlboro cigarette, crossed his legs, and drew himself back before bringing up his problem. At last, he said, "Doc, I'm having trouble with the boy who's dating my daughter."

Relief swelled over me when I realized that all he wanted was advice on his daughter's love life. He had three very attractive tall blond daughters, and the eldest had just turned seventeen. The concern in his face told me that he was very troubled about the girl's well-being and was looking to me for some serious consultation. I don't know why he had chosen me—probably just because I was the closest available human at the time he needed to get this off his chest.

The problem was that the boyfriend was very disrespectful to Mr. Stanley, not abiding by the dating rules that he had set down. When Mr. Stanley told the young man to have his daughter home by a certain time, the boy said he could do as he pleased, then informed Mr. Stanley that he couldn't touch him and that he would bring her home when he was good and ready. My first thought was that I never would have dreamed of arguing with this protective Nordic father when I was a kid. In fact, I would have referred to him as "sir" and always had his daughter home at least a half hour early. It was unfathomable that a high school kid would mouth off to this impressive figure.

We discussed the possibility of burying the boy in the backyard but decided against it due to possible prison terms. After tossing around several different torture ideas, Mr. Stanley decided that it might be best if he called Romeo's parents first. I suggested that the effect could be greater if he knocked on their door himself, and he seemed happy with that plan. An appreciative smile broke loose under his sandy mustache hairs as he shook my hand vigorously enough to give me tennis elbow. "Thanks, Doc," he said. "I really appreciate your time. I'll go and see them this evening." "No problem—anytime," I replied, returning his smile. Meanwhile, I was thinking, I'm sure glad I'm not that boy's parents.

My pickup sped down the Stanleys' winding driveway through the shimmering aspen trees, and I felt satisfaction that I had been able to be there not only for the sick horse but also for the worried father. He'd actually figured it out on his own; he'd just needed someone to run things by.

Developing relationships with my clients has always been an enjoyable part of practice for me, which often puts me in a position of being a sounding board. Many medical doctors and their patients complain that the human element has been removed from medicine due to the problems caused by insurance companies, HMOs, and liability suits. Marion deals with this balancing act daily in her practice as a physician's assistant. She tries to do a good job, spend enough time with the patients, and still be able to attend to all the people who have to be seen each day. By closing time, she is exhausted, both mentally and physically. Maybe veterinary medicine isn't that tough after all.

I have watched families go through good times and bad times and have watched their children grow up. I've spent late nights putting the family dog back together while swapping life stories with the owner. But even after all these experiences, I am still amazed by what people will tell their veterinarian. Sometimes you realize that a conversation is headed in a bad direction and you try desperately to change the subject, but you can't quite pull the client back from the edge. Some people are just determined that they are going to subject you to the gory details, like it or not. Often these stories relate to the client's own medical problems, which may be completely inappropriate for me to hear. The opposite happens to Marion. When her patients hear she is married to a veterinarian, they almost always run their pets' problems by her. "Well, I don't mean to be looking for free advice, but my cat . . ." At least animal questions aren't usually embarrassing or overly personal.

On one particular occasion, I was checking a mare for fertility issues. With the help of a large speculum, I was performing a thorough reproductive exam. It was at this point that the client chimed in with some experiences of her own. Joni May was a small-framed woman in her late thirties, with fiery red hair and bright blue eyes. I had seen her only a couple of times before, once when her basset hound ate an entire giant solid-chocolate bunny on Easter morning. She had been very easy to deal with and extremely happy that I had saved her dog from death by chocolate. Excessive caffeine from large amounts of chocolate can actually cause a dog to have a heart attack. We took care of the chocolate-loving pup, and I had been on good terms with her ever since.

But on this day, she seemed confused about the fact that she was talking to a health-care provider for animals only. She started to tell me how she and her husband had a hard time having children. Delving into the extensive testing that she had been through, she rambled on with all the vivid details of the medical visits, then looked to me as if I might have some ideas that they hadn't tried yet. I wanted to put my index fingers in my ears and hum so as not to hear any more. I guess my discomfort showed because she said, "Well, you are a doctor, after all, aren't you?" Then, before I could stop her, she went into her husband's fertility history—just what every man wants discussed with a relative stranger. All I could think was how embarrassed he would be to hear this conversation. Finally, she took a long breath, giving me enough time to interrupt. I explained that I had experience only with animals and was not really qualified to give advice concerning humans. Can you imagine explaining this one to the judge in the malpractice hearing? "But, sir, it works for horses."

Fortunately, this reasoning seemed to satisfy her, and she switched to safer topics, such as the septic tank problems they were having. I finally was able get a uterine culture from the mare and found the source of her reproductive problems. Mrs. May, on the other hand, I sent back to her gynecologist. I wonder if she asked the doctor about her horse.

Scalpel, Please

If I were to associate the surgical part of my practice with a human medical specialty, it would
have to be obstetrics, in that the need for surgery,
especially in large animals, rarely occurs during
office hours. I can commiserate with physicians who, bleary-eyed,
crawl from their warm beds to attend to the needs of women in the
throes of labor. But at least they tend to do their work in the fluorescent glow of the hospital delivery room, coming in to don the sterile
gloves in the nick of time to catch the emerging head. This, after the
obstetrical nurse has called the anesthesiologist, monitored the newly
administered epidural, and placed the sterile drape. In the case of
a cesarean section, the patient is whisked away to the surgical suite
and attended to. God willing, all goes well and mother and child are
reunited, face-to-face, with either form of delivery.

In mixed-animal practice, surgical procedures are not as tidy as
one might desire. I've always imagined performing surgery on a horse

or cow and yelling out "Clamp!" like a medical doctor on a hospital television show, then having some smiling nurse actually hand me one. Much to my disappointment, this is nothing more than a fantasy in the world of veterinary surgery. I'm usually lucky if I can find the appropriate instrument at all. I've grown accustomed to holding a dirty flashlight in my teeth as I rifle through my sterile surgical pack in a dimly lit barn.

I have been on more calls than I care to remember when my fingers were so cold I couldn't feel them while suturing a cut horse or bringing a calf into the world through an incision in the mother's side. During these situations, the anesthetic is also the veterinarian's responsibility, so no one else can be blamed if the correct level of sedation is not achieved. Too little can result in a swift kick to the head, and too much can make for a very disappointed owner, due to dangerous results for the animal. This is one of the reasons I always work very hard to avoid having to perform a cesarean section on an animal, encouraging the baby to come out the natural route if possible. On one particular January evening in the Colorado mountains, however, this just wasn't going to happen.

I was called out to a small ranch in a picturesque valley at the base of Mount Evans. I had been practicing in the region for only about a year, but the Cunninghams were already good clients. They had several horses, a pack of dogs of assorted sizes, and about ten cows. The cattle were Mr. Cunningham's project, and he had just enough of them, in his mind, to call himself a rancher. In real life, he was an engineer who traveled a lot as a consultant. He was the tall, dark, silent type, who, instead of speaking, preferred to peer over his glasses in a mistrusting way. I always felt he never fully agreed with my diagnoses, producing more leering whenever I handed him the bill. His wife was left to handle the animals and ride herd over their six children whenever Mr. Cunningham was traveling for work. Fortunately, they had a beautiful log home—which would have fit well in a fancy resort town like Aspen—to kennel the dogs and children.

Mrs. Cunningham's name was Lizzy, and she was a transplant from Southern California who came during the period when it appeared the whole state was migrating to Colorado. She seemed to love her life here in the Rockies and, unlike her husband, was extremely easy to deal with. She was always happy to see me and acted as if she got the best out of every day. A willing work partner in life for her husband, she didn't mind getting her hands dirty or getting the occasional horse or cow tail in the face.

She did have one interesting trait she carried with her from her California days that she just couldn't seem to shake, and that was her manner of dressing. No matter what the weather was like or how muddy the corral, she always wore her designer outfits. I looked forward to seeing what she would come out of the house in. Her wardrobe usually included designer jeans, an Ann Taylor top, and flip-flops. In these, she would head down to the barn lot to wrestle a horse or cow. She was a great help, never backing away from a beast in need, yet somehow managing to keep her attire perfectly clean. My clothes would usually be covered with blood and fecal material after caring for an animal, yet she was still clean enough to have tea with the First Lady. Lizzy and I had a good working relationship, so when she paged me on this night, I was a little disappointed to hear that it would be Mr. Cunningham helping me deliver the calf this time.

He met me in the field near a grove of ponderosa pines. The cow was lying down in the snow, straining with labor and not making any progress. Two larger-than-normal hooves stuck out behind her, but there was no sign of a head or snout. Mr. Cunningham nodded to me, allowing his glasses to slide down his nose. I stared at his chiseled face and then got to work.

I put on the traditional long latex glove and slathered it with lubricant. Next came one of my least favorite things: kneeling in the snow and not knowing how long it would be before I could put on a dry pair of pants. Within seconds, the melting snow penetrated my jeans and the cold crept in. Thrusting my hand into the cow, I could feel the moist nose of the calf at the far end of the birth canal. Then came that sensation that always makes my heart jump—it tried to suck on my finger. The calf was still alive, but it was a long way from entering the world.

It wasn't long before Mr. Cunningham was growing very impatient, kicking the snow about with his feet. I wanted to say, Will someone please remove this man and send him to the father's waiting room? I was still kneeling there in the snow as Mr. Cunningham began clearing his throat. Eventually, he spoke. "Well, let's get on with it. Can't you get the calf out?" I didn't respond right away. Having your arm wedged between a calf's skull and a cow's pelvis tends to make you a little less accepting of criticism or advice than normal, I've discovered. From my vantage point beside the cow, with my jeans now stiffly frozen, I wondered what I'd been thinking when I decided to become a veterinarian. I was pretty sure the business majors I went to college with were tucked into bed by now and weren't staring at Mr. Cunningham, wondering what to tell him. Oh, to have a desk, a 401(k) plan with a percentage supplemented by the company, and clean shoes—that's what I was thinking about to keep my mind off the sting of the snow on my knees.

But I gazed up at the stars in the clear Colorado sky and the moonlight bouncing off the snow on Mount Evans, reminding myself that it wasn't such a bad place to be after all. Then Mr. Cunningham's throat clearing cut the crisp air—just what I needed to snap me back to the task before me. "The calf is too big. It's going to have to come out the side," I told him.

Mr. Cunningham appeared to be shocked. "What on earth do you mean?" he responded, wide-eyed. This was the most emotion he had ever shown in my presence. He was the kind of man who tried to act as if he knew a lot about livestock, although truly he had a sparse acquaintance with the subject. This small ranch was a hobby for him, allowing him to talk like a cattleman when the flight was long or the conversation lulled.

"We'll have to perform a cesarean section on the cow right here or we're going to lose them both." As I heard myself say these words, it sunk in how much work was ahead of me. The prospect of opening up his cow and removing a calf in the middle of a snow-covered field silenced Mr. Cunningham. I was also sure he noticed my use of the word *we,* implying that he would be helping.

"I don't know, I just don't know," he repeated. I knew I had him on the run now. The superiority had left his voice, and he sank to my level.

"Well, we don't really have any choice, do we? They'll both die without the operation." He finally shrugged his shoulders, admitting that he was no longer calling the shots—nature was.

I dragged the surgery pack out of the truck and produced a syringeful of tranquilizer to make the cow's life easier. The sting of the needle stimulated her to get to her feet, so we tied her head to a tree in order to keep her around for the operation. An old stump that stuck out just above the snow would have to act as an instrument stand, I decided, and the moon, along with my headlights, would substitute as surgical lights. Next, I injected the local anesthetic into the cow's side and clipped away the hair. With very few species of domestic animals could you pull off this surgery in the middle of a meadow, but fortunately cows seem to tolerate it beautifully.

One of my professors used to joke that one could spit into a cow's abdomen and it wouldn't affect the end result, but none of us ever tried it. I sterilized the surgical site with a soapy Betadine-soaked gauze pad and was just ready to drape it off, when Mr. Cunningham thrust his dirty hand right smack in the middle of the freshly scrubbed area.

"Is this the spot where we're going to cut?" he asked. Now it was my turn to leer.

"Yes, it is, but let's not touch it again," I mumbled. He drew back out of the light, and I commenced with another vigorous cleansing.

Finally, I pulled on the stiff, cold surgery gloves and made the incision. Warm blood oozed onto my hands, temporarily thawing my frozen fingertips. I cut quickly through the muscle layers, exposing the uterus. By now, the cow had dug through the snow and was chomping on the dead grass below. After the sedative kicked in, she was totally oblivious to the fact that she was a patient.

Mr. Cunningham, who had been watching from afar, was about to become an active participant. "Please put on those extra gloves on the end of my tailgate and give me a hand," I said. I could tell he wanted to give me one of his looks, but he abstained. He donned the gloves and helped me pull the uterus through the incision just enough to get the calf out without allowing fluid to seep back into the cow's abdomen. He held it in place while I incised the uterus and pulled out the calf. Its coat was slimy and matted, and its ears lay flat against its head. There were no signs of life.

I placed him on my tailgate and began trying to stimulate him to take his first breaths. Normally, the cow would have stimulated the calf with a good thorough washing with her rough tongue. Our mother remained comfortably numb, however, detached from her primal instincts, thanks to the anesthesia.

After a good rubdown with a towel and a couple of handy pine needles stuck up his nose to stimulate breathing, the lifeless form at last shook his head and began to breathe. Normally, this would have been a celebratory event for me, but snowflakes had begun to fall. Layers of cow abdomen awaited closure, and Mr. Cunningham was getting grumpy, holding a cooling uterus in his own cooling hands. I closed the womb, pushed it back into the warm abdomen, and put him to work drying off the calf. A veterinarian I had worked with as a student once gave me sage advice: "Always give the tough ones a job to do to keep them out of your hair!" Mr. Cunningham got to work, rubbing the calf with dry hay.

The snow came down harder, like some kind of cruel prank, as I sutured. Toward the end, I was blowing the snow out of the incision between every suture and digging through three inches of snow to find my instruments. At last, the final skin suture was placed, and the cow hadn't kicked me yet. Thankfully, the sedation remained effective until the very last minute.

To give the newborn a better chance, I squeezed some warm milk from the mother's udder into a large syringe. The sedation was completely worn off by now, and since she wasn't dairy cow used to being milked, she immediately shot out a back leg like a piston near my head.

The first milk an animal produces upon giving birth is packed with carbohydrates and proteins. This fluid, known as colostrum, is the closest thing to magic I have ever seen. Squirting it down even a very weak youngster can literally bring it back to life, and this little guy was no exception. Within a minute of feeding the calf this gift of life, he shook himself off and stood up, looking for more. We untied

Mom, and the two ran off into the storm. I knocked the snow off all my tools and packed them away in the truck, planning to clean up the mess the next morning in the warmth of the clinic. I informed Mr. Cunningham that the sutures would need to come out in two weeks, then opened the truck door to make my escape. Just then, I heard the throat clearing start up again. I thought this was it—that he was actually going to thank me—but instead he grunted, "You forgot this," and handed me a blood-soaked towel. Then he vanished into the night.

I was wet, freezing, and wishing the hot air would start coming out of the vents in my pickup. I think my heart was even becoming a little frozen as I sat there, wondering what career I should try next. Then a steaming mug in the cup holder caught my attention. It was filled with hot chocolate, and beside me on the passenger seat was a bag holding a dozen still-warm chocolate-chip cookies. Mrs. Cunningham had sneaked down with these treats while I was finishing up the surgery. I gulped the cocoa and inhaled the cookies. By the time I pulled in our driveway, I found Marion had left a light on, and the cocoa had brought my body back to its normal temperature. It was enough to make me think that veterinary practice wasn't so bad after all, and that I could stick with it a little longer.

Bosley

The first time I saw Bosley and Mr. Eichler, I was absolutely astonished. I had heard of these situations, but I myself had never seen one so dramatic. Mr. Eichler and his basset hound, Bosley, looked amazingly alike. Mr. Eichler had the same droopy eyes and sad expression. His cheeks were saggy with age and his nose was larger than normal. However, his ears, though larger than those of most humans, did not hang below his face. Mr. Eichler was a retired college professor, and he dressed the part. The bald portion of his head was covered with a flat hat, set off with a checkered bow tie. He was a man of few words, speaking only when necessary. Bosley had an appointment for a toenail trim. Now, basset hounds are not known for tolerating manicures well, and Bosley was no exception.

It took both Christie and me to get Bosley from the floor to the exam table. He may have had short legs, but the rest of his body was thick and solid. We strained and puffed just to get him onto the Formica surface of the exam table, nearly inducing my first hernia.

Up to now, the mild-mannered Bosley had been more than cooperative, but when Christie rolled him on his side, his saggy lips curled, exposing large canine teeth. I held his front right leg firmly below the paw and began whittling away at the first nail. Like other bassets' nails, his were thick and heavy, made for digging holes to find rodents. Bosley's objections started escalating as I continued knocking back the claws. He attempted pulling his leg away from my grasp while at the same time snapping at my hand with his pearly whites. Christie tightened her grip on him, leaning over the table and putting some of her body weight on his chest. Bosley responded by twisting around until he got himself onto his back. This move put us at a major disadvantage. Christie had completely lost her hold, and Bosley took control of the situation. He scraped my arms and hands with his digging tools while snapping at Christie. On his back, he was like an upside-down alligator. Mr. Eichler snickered, then looked embarrassed. "I'm sorry, he is always like this. He's the best dog I've ever had, but when it comes to this nail-trimming business, he just turns into a little monster." There was no winning this battle now. We backed off and Bosley righted himself. Mr. Eichler apologized profusely. "I haven't been completely honest with you. Bosley and I have been to several other veterinarians for attempted nail trims, and it never ends well. We've even been asked to leave." This caused Christie to flash me a raised eyebrow. That look actually meant, Let's figure out a way to get them out of here before things get really bad. Yet Mr. Eichler seemed like such a nice guy and Bosley seemed to be a great dog, except for the nail issues. Some owners are averse to using sedatives for such minor procedures, and understandably so. With any medication, there is always that slight possibility of an undesirable side effect, but the options were not plentiful in this case. I thought for a minute, then brought up sedation. "I think the best thing to do for Bosley's sake and ours is to use just a little sedative." Now the ball was in Mr. Eichler's court. He pondered for a few seconds, twisting his mouth while staring at his smiling pooch. "Well, we have turned down drugs before, but Bosley's long nails are really beginning to scratch up the floor." He lifted his hat, rubbing his head. "If you think we can do it with just a little, let's do it." I nodded, heading into the treatment room for some mood-altering medication, and Christie scowled at me. She knew what I was trying to ignore: A little sedation was not likely going to do it. As I pulled up a tad of the drug, I knew I should be filling the syringe right to the brim, but I could not betray Mr. Eichler's trust.

Returning to the exam room, I found Christie still glaring. Mr. Eichler was fidgeting, and Bosley was obviously wondering what else we had in our bag of tricks. "Now, you're just giving him a smidgen, right?" Mr. Eichler made one last check. I reassured him, saying, "The smallest dose for his size, I assure you." I held the syringe up to show him and he squinted to see if I actually had anything in it. Christie reluctantly held off the vein and I administered the minute dosage. Sometimes, if you are very lucky, an underdose of a sedative will be just enough to take the edge off of an upset animal. They may still require some restraint, but it allows one to avoid an outright wrestling match. This was the response I was hoping for—the one that Christie was sure we were not going to get. After a couple minutes of all three of us staring at Bosley, he appeared to become a little groggy. His eyes seemed very slightly glazed over and his breathing slowed some. The fact that Mr. Eicher asked, "He is going to be okay, isn't he?" made me feel Bosley's relaxation was more than just the product of my hopeful imagination.

I compromised with Christie to keep her on my team: I would hold Bosley and she would trim his nails. I coaxed Bosley onto his side, holding his left front leg with my left hand and draping my left forearm over his neck. Christie went for the first nail and I increased the pressure on Bosley's neck slightly. He struggled for a couple of seconds, then relaxed. The fight decreased with every nail, ending completely by the second paw. The "edge off" theory had actually worked. Bosley fell into a relaxed daze, giving in to the ultimate basset humiliation.

Mr. Eichler was elated and thanked us profusely on his way out the door. The last thing I heard him say was, "You've got a new client." Was that a good thing? Christie didn't think so. "You got lucky that time; it won't be that way the next time," she told me.

Fortunately, she was wrong. Bosley started coming in every two months for a nail trim. We went through the same routine every time, and every time Bosley submitted a little more quickly. The day came when Bosley's visits were not dreaded at all. We began to enjoy seeing this low rider come through the door with Mr. Eichler in tow and being greeted by Bosley's unrelenting tail wag.

I had gotten to know Mr. Eichler fairly well over the exam table. He'd told me of his years of teaching college English in the Northeast and how he missed those days. "I often wish I was still teaching," he would say. "People need purpose and a place to go when they get up in the morning." He was the type of person who had wrapped himself around his career and hadn't had time for much else. For Mr. Eichler, dedication to career seemed to have made retirement an especially hard adjustment. He never mentioned a Mrs. Eichler, but he wore a gold band on the appropriate finger, making us wonder if he was widowed. He appeared to enjoy his outings to the clinic with Bosley. He would often linger in the waiting room afterward to talk with Lorraine about how fast-paced things were now or how people today did not use proper English.

Everything clicked along with Bosley and Mr. Eichler for quite some time, but then one nippy fall day we got a call that Bosley was not doing well. He was lethargic and not eating much. Not at all normal for an animal that Mr. Eichler had previously referred to as "a vacuum cleaner with legs—close to the ground so he can't miss anything."

The car pulled in, and when Mr. Eichler helped Bosley out of the car, the dog could barely walk. Then Mr. Eichler ran around to the other side to open the door for another person. There *was* a Mrs. Eichler! Out stepped a very properly dressed woman in her late sixties. Mr Eichler held the door for her, as he probably had for almost half a century, and she headed for the office—without assisting Bosley. She stormed in, establishing her position from the start. "I don't know what he sees in that old dog. I had many more pressing errands to run today."

Mr. Eichler opened the door and Bosley staggered through it in front of him. "I'm very concerned, Doctor. He seems to be going downhill fast. Oh, and this is my wife," he said as he nodded his head in her direction. "We just met," I replied. "Now let's take a look at Bosley." We got him up on the table and I started to examine him. "Well, what is the problem?" Mrs. Eichler asked. Mr. Eichler's head dropped even lower, and I just proceeded with my exam. Bosley's respiratory rate was faster than normal and his gums were slightly pale. Even the whites around his eyes were more pale than usual. His temperature was normal, even though he objected to my method of taking it. Bosley showed all the classic signs of anemia, but I had no idea what was causing it. "Bosley is a little anemic." I spoke directly to Mr. Eichler. Then I said the words that make all owners think we are just buying time. "We need to run some tests." Mrs. Eichler responded by saying, "How much is that going to cost?" Mr. Eichler looked me in the eye and nodded his head. We pulled some blood and sent Bosley on his way. "We'll talk first thing in the morning, once the blood tests have come back," I said to Mr. Eichler as he was walking out the door. "Try to get him to eat something tonight. Maybe some treats or something he really likes." I gave him a reassuring pat on the shoulder, sending him on his way.

The blood-work results were waiting for me on the fax machine when I got to the office the next day. Bosley was officially anemic. His red blood cells were markedly decreased, but every other test was normal. All organ-function tests were on target and there were no changes in white blood cell counts that would indicate an infection. Even the platelets, which participate in blood clotting, were present in totally normal amounts.

I called Mr. Eichler, explaining the results. "Doctor, I was just getting ready to call you. Bosley passed some very dark stool this morning and he's getting more depressed." "Well, let's bring him in and take another look," I replied. "Come in right away and bring the stool sample with you." Now I was going to have to figure out what was wrong without the help of an easy diagnosis from blood work.

Bosley and Mr. Eichler showed up without their "better half" this time. Mr. Eichler immediately presented me with a clear plastic bag full of everything that had come out of Bosley's colon over the last twelve hours. Christie checked the sample for blood, and it came back positive. Bosley was losing blood into his intestines. On examination, he had a slight amount of bleeding from the gums. Bosley was moving in a bad direction, and I had no idea how to stop it. My boss was out hiking that day, so there was no way to consult with him. I was getting really close to referring Bosley to a big hospital in Denver, a responsible move for a young veterinarian with no clue about a case. I knew I was missing something, but I just couldn't put my finger on it. I asked Mr. Eichler to take Bosley and to sit in the waiting room for a few minutes, then I retreated into the back office. I pulled the ten-pound volume of *Small Animal Medicine* off the shelf and dusted it off. Under "Canine Anemia" I found several diseases that I had already ruled out with the blood work. I was just about to slam the book shut and send them down the road. Then the words nearly popped off the page and grabbed me by the throat: *warfarin poisoning*. Why had I not thought of it earlier—rat poisoning? Back in the waiting room, I questioned Mr. Eichler. "Have you put out any rat poisoning recently? I'm concerned that Bosley may have gotten into some." He replied, "As a matter of fact, I have, just a couple weeks ago. My wife saw a mouse in the house when it first started to get cold, so I put some down in the crawl space under the house." With Bosley's genetic predisposition for digging and rooting around, it was not hard to imagine him forcing his way into the crawl space and sniffing out the poison for a snack. Mr. Eichler called his wife to ask her to check under the house. After lots of convincing, she gave in. Sure enough, the wooden door to the crawl space had been forced open. "Bosley dug out of his pen a few days ago. I'll bet that is when he got into it," Mr. Eichler said triumphantly.

The warfarin in the poison had caused a deficiency in vitamin K, important in the blood-clotting process. Thus, the treatment was to supplement vitamin K. Bosley went home after a large injection of vitamin K and a month's worth of the same in tablet form. Mr. Eichler listened closely to my instructions, nodding his head to let me know he understood. If there was anyone who would follow the instructions to a tee, it would be Mr. Eicher, I knew. "We need to get him back in again in a couple days to make sure he is not still losing red blood cells. If the count gets too low, we may have to do a blood transfusion," I informed him. "So you can make an appointment with Lorraine now if you like." The look on Mr. Eichler's face made me feel that I had said something wrong. He hesitated for a second, then said, "I'll call back when I get home." After the door shut behind them, Lorraine chuckled. "He has to get permission from his wife." Sure enough, within the hour he called back to set it up.

In two days, the pair was back in and we took another blood sample from Bosley, who was just happy we were not trimming his nails. The count had not gone any lower. "It looks like Bosley is already stabilizing; he must not have eaten very much of the poison," I said, happy to be giving Mr. Eichler this news. "We should probably check it a couple more times just to be sure, but he seems to be doing well." "Oh, thank you so much, Doctor," he said with the happiest expression I had seen from him yet. "I don't know what I would have done without him. He is my best friend in the world." He shook my hand vigorously. We saw Bosley a few more times for blood tests and he continued to improve.

Almost three months later, Bosley, Mr. Eichler, and Mrs. Eichler were all in the waiting room. Bosley was obviously doing well. I assumed that Bosley was in for his regular nail-trimming visit. But why is Mrs. Eichler here? I wondered. She never came along for something that benign, and she had a medium-size pet carrier beside her. They all paraded into the exam room, Mrs. Eicher dragging the carrier. "Doctor," Mr. Eichler said. "We're here for more than just a nail trim today. The day that Bosley broke out of his pen and got into the poison, he also made a trip to the neighbors'. "Well, the neighbors have a female rottweiler." At the same time, Mrs. Eichler reached into the carrier and produced a puppy. It had the black-and-brown markings of a rottweiler, along with the distinct long body and stubby wrinkled legs of a basset hound. There were five puppies in all. Now, all puppies are cute, these included, yet they did look like some type of genetic aberration. "We're here to drop off Bosley for a neuter and five expensive puppy shots." Mrs. Eichler announced. "We are holding up our end of this paternity situation." The Eichlers had made a deal with the owners of the female that they would have the shots done and help to find homes for the puppies. The other part of this neighborly agreement was that Bosley would have to be "taken care of" so that this would never happen again. Mr. Eichler looked as if we were neutering him instead of his dog. He stroked Bosley's back, telling him all would be okay. Finally, he gave me his usual nod to tell me to go ahead. "He'll be fine," I assured him. We'll trim his nails while he's under."

The surgery went fine, and Mr. Eichler was waiting at the door to pick him up at eight o'clock the next morning. Elated to see that Bosley seemed no worse for wear, he thanked us all and took off to buy Bosley a postsurgical hamburger.

Bosley's offspring all found good homes, and some began to trickle into the clinic for care. Then one day, a lady showed up with one of them, requesting a nail trim. "I tried to cut them myself, but he turned into a real monster," she complained. Christie and I just stood there dumbfounded. Neither one of us had thought about this possibility: an animal who shared Bosley's disdain of toe trims but had the strength of a rottweiler. This was not going to be fun.

Collateral

Most of us who go into veterinary medicine look forward to helping sick and injured animals and don't think initially about things like getting paid or how to deal with delinquent accounts. Most clients are really good about paying, but every so often an uncomfortable situation arises concerning a bill. A few unpaid bills here and there don't seem like they'd be that big a deal, but they add up over time. What people forget is that we have not only worked hard to save their pets or livestock but may have used expensive medications that have to be replaced. And to top things off, the staff likes to get paid occasionally. If practicing for free becomes the rule rather than the exception, bankruptcy and foreclosure are not far behind, which means that the veterinarian will no longer be around to look after the welfare of the animals.

Most veterinarians try to prevent this problem by coming up with innovative ways to ensure they get paid. Some practitioners turn to collection agencies. While I've found these can be used as a last-ditch effort, what has worked well for me is taking collateral. If clients leave behind an item that they want back badly enough, they almost always seem to come up with the money. Being a rather nonconfrontational person, I can find it hard to bring up the subject of payment, let alone collateral, but it has become a necessary evil. An interesting aspect of taking people's material belongings in hopes they will eventually want them back is seeing what they consider valuable. Over the years, I have collected everything from leather jackets to diamond broaches, and fortunately I've traded nearly all of the items for payment of clients' bills.

One summer morning, Marion and I were halfway through our Wheaties and the *Today* show when an emergency page came through from a Mrs. Gordon. "I'm a little embarrassed," she began, "but my cat, Tom, had a kitten about an hour ago and is straining as if more are coming. We just thought Tom was getting a little overweight. I guess we'll have to rename her." She continued to tell me that she had not been a client of ours before and that she had no money right then to pay for our services. Her husband had already gone to work, she said, but he would be able to take care of the bill on his way home.

By this point in my career, I had heard all the lines at least twice and was becoming a little skeptical of humankind. I thought for a couple of moments and decided to hedge my bets a little. "Do you think that maybe you could bring in some collateral until your husband can come by?" I asked.

Now it was her turn to hesitate "Well . . . I guess I could come up with something. Yes, I know just the thing."

"Great," I replied, always hopeful. "I'll meet you at the clinic and we'll see what we can do for old Tom." I hung up the phone, wondering what "valuable" item she would show up with.

It was one of those mornings that, although it sounds sappy, makes you just glad to be alive. The sky was azure blue, without a single cloud to break it up, a treat that Colorado seems to supply on a fairly regular basis. It was well before office hours, so I took a seat behind the front counter of the clinic to wait for Mrs. Gordon. I was beginning to bob my head a little when her custom van roared up the driveway, sliding to a stop at the last minute. Within seconds, she popped out the door on the driver's side, a cat carrier in her left hand, a baby in the crook of her arm, and a .30-06 high-powered hunting rifle in her right hand—an interesting choice for collateral. I hurried to hold the door open for her, as a man with any sense would do for a woman packing that much heat. She laid the rifle down beside the straining cat on the exam table. I quickly toted the weapon off to the back office, just in case things didn't go quite as planned.

Tom's one live kitten was already enjoying a buffet of milk all to herself, but no more siblings were appearing. I examined the birth canal, hoping to find a head or a tail to get hold of and slip out into the world, but no such luck. At this point, we had two choices: a cesarean section or an injection to encourage the cat to push the kittens out the natural way. Most veterinarians choose the conservative route first, so I reached for the bottle of oxytocin. Pitocin, as it is known in human medicine, causes the uterus to start contracting again even when the organ has given up from hours of labor.

Eventually, the injection kicked in, and Tom started to become uncomfortable from the straining. This time, my examination revealed a tiny white tail and a pair of mouselike pink rear feet. After putting on some sterile gloves, I was able to get one of the feet between my index finger and my second finger and began to tug at the reluctant little animal. Pulling on the leg with only two fingers got to be tedious quickly, yet the kitten seemed to get a little closer to coming into the world with every try, so I kept after it. Just when my fingers were starting to cramp, the kitten popped out into the world like a cork from a wine bottle.

"Is it alive?" Mrs. Gordon whispered. This was the question I always heard the second any newborn came into the world. The miracle of birth has never worn off for me, no matter what species it is, but the elation is stifled when there is a question of life. This tiny feline wasn't moving, and his tongue had a tinge of blue. I placed him on his side, cleaned the mucus out of his mouth, and pumped gently on his chest with my fingers. After several pumps, oxygenated blood returned to the tongue, and the infant cat began to wiggle. It coughed a couple of times, shook its fuzzy head, and started moving toward the milk bar.

While I was resuscitating the kitten, four more fuzz balls had appeared on the table. The breech one had been holding up the show, and once he was out of the road, the rest found their own way. Now Mrs. Gordon really had her hands full: seven new babies, including the human one.

I helped her pack them up and get them all back in the van—just in time, as it turned out, because someone needed a clean diaper and other clients would be coming in soon. Just before slamming the rusting van door, she called out, "My husband will be in this evening to settle up."

"I'll believe it when I see it," I mumbled after the door was safely closed.

Lorraine, our receptionist, walked in as the Gordon clan pulled onto the highway. She turned up her nose and began cleaning up the exam table. "You had an early start," she said with a sneer. She always appeared to get great enjoyment out of my long hours. In reality, she was more valuable to the practice than an inexperienced veterinarian like me, and she knew it. There were innumerable young veterinarians who were eager to practice in Colorado, but a good, organized receptionist was hard to find.

The rest of the day was rather uneventful—a couple of elective surgeries and a lame llama in the afternoon. We were just about ready to close the doors at 7:00 P.M., hours we kept for the convenience of those who could make it in only after their workday was finished. Christie was trying to get away for another "big date," and Lorraine was calling home to see what she needed to pick up on the way.

I was beginning to wonder what the rifle in the back was worth, when a pickup tore up the driveway. It was one of those souped-up varieties with oversize tires and silhouettes of provocative women on the mud flaps. It even had a gun rack in the rear window, but the gun was missing. The clinic door flew open and a large man stepped in, looking a little agitated. He had a mullet haircut and an orange baseball cap with a buck deer on the bill. By the look of things, he didn't like wasting money on shaving razors, maybe saving it instead for beer.

"My wife said she left my rifle here, and I'm here to get it back," he began without even saying hello.

I squelched the urge to run back to the office, grab the rifle, give it back to him without asking for any form of payment, and then apologize and hide behind my desk until he left. Instead, I managed to hold my ground. "Thanks for coming in, Mr. Gordon," I said, trying to sound both casual and cheerful. "We were able to save all of Tom's kittens, and Tom, too."

He hesitated for a minute, then spoke again. "But we thought that Tom was . . ." I replied, "I know, but that's an easy mistake to make. We even confuse young kittens here at the clinic occasionally."

His expression began to soften; maybe he was thinking of his baby daughter playing with the squirming newborn kittens at home. "I guess I would miss that old cat if anything happened to him . . . or her. It's just that the rifle was my father's; he died last year, and it's the only thing I have left that was his."

Nodding sheepishly, I went to get the rifle while Mr. Gordon wrote out a check for the bill and gave it to Lorraine. I felt somewhat remorseful about having taken his rifle hostage. Evidently, I should have had more faith. He thanked us profusely, then headed for home, his keepsake restored. I sent Lorraine on her way. As I locked up, I thought about what a pity it is that a few people's dishonesty leads to dilemmas like this for the rest of us.

Contagious

I can't understand what this man is talking about," the receptionist said, pointing to the phone, on which the hold light was flashing. "It's something about a cat and maybe hair loss. You try to talk to him."

When I picked up the phone, the voice on the other end spoke in a syrupy southern accent that sounded almost alien. "How y'all doing, Doc?" was nearly all I could decipher. I did catch something about his cat, intermixed with a series of words that were completely unrecognizable. I returned the phone to the receptionist and told her to have the fellow bring in his pet at three o'clock.

My boss was gone on vacation that week and we had a relief vet filling in. With such a big demand for relief veterinarians in recent years, many practitioners make their living this way, working at a number of different clinics so the more permanent fixtures can take some time off—vacation time is a precious commodity in any veterinary practice. Dr. Sally was a fine small-animal practitioner and was also excellent with the owners. She took her work very seriously and cared deeply for her patients, but humor was not one of her strong suits. This slightly intense attitude made it hard not to pull the occasional prank on her, and Christie snickered when I suggested that Dr. Sally should see the cat from Dixie that afternoon. Dr. Sally was originally from upper New Jersey, and we knew that trying to get a feline history filtered through a deep southern accent would frustrate her no end.

I caught her coming out of an exam room with a small dog tucked under her arm. She had just spent the last half hour convincing an owner that her precious miniature poodle would not expire if he stayed overnight for some much-needed dental work. Dr. Sally reluctantly nodded her head when I explained the situation involving the client I wanted her to see for me. "What do you mean, you couldn't understand the man? Didn't he tell you what was wrong with the cat?"

"I think they may be from out of town; he had a little bit of an accent," I responded. "Unfortunately, I have another appointment coming in about the same time." She sighed and agreed to work the cat into her schedule.

A few hours later, I noticed a thirty-something couple sitting patiently in the waiting room. The husband was dressed in a gray work shirt and matching pants, with the insignia of a local trucking company over the left breast pocket. He held his matching gray cap in his lap; it was stained with perspiration around the brim. His wife, a robust woman, wore a clean paisley dress covered above the waist with the familiar blue vest issued by a well-known big-box store. Between them was a white pillow slip tied in a knot at the opening. Something seemed to be in it, and occasionally it moved like a ghost in an old Scooby-Doo cartoon.

People use many different forms of containment to bring cats into the vet's office. I have seen cats confined in everything from duffel bags to elaborate cat carriers, but one of my favorites has always been the basic pillow slip. Upset cats seem to grow mellow in this converted bedding, and it is just porous enough to allow air transfer, though I don't believe pillowcases are sanctioned by the American Veterinary Medical Association. I had a feeling that these were the people I had attempted to speak to earlier. Sure enough, they headed in to see Dr. Sally with a "How y'all doing today?"

Henry and Missy McCoy seemed to respond fairly well to Dr. Sally's direct approach. I could hear the conversation outside the other door in the treatment area. Dr. Sally began with the usual questions about medical history. "How long has Mr. Biscuits had these missing patches of hair? Does he scratch the bare spots?"

A couple of hems and haws came from the other side of the door, followed by a "Could you say that again?" The McCoys hung on every word, as if Sally was about to make an earth-shattering scientific discovery.

Our visiting veterinarian then reached under the exam table, slid open the drawer, and produced a black light. This tool was not to light up an Elvis painting but to cause the suspected fungus on the skin of the cat to fluoresce and amaze the audience. Such glowing patches are always impressive, but Dr. Sally had not yet conveyed the reason for this strange sight to Mr. Biscuits' owners. Finally, the McCoys couldn't stand it anymore, and Henry spoke up. "Do you have any idea what it is, Doc?"

Dr. Sally snapped back, "Well, Mr. Biscuits has a bad case of ringworm." The pride of an unquestionable diagnosis oozed from under the door, outside of which I was shamelessly eavesdropping.

Mrs. McCoy gasped. "How on earth do the worms get under the

skin?" Sally then explained that ringworm did not involve any kind of a worm and was actually caused by a fungus.

As she began to shave the infected areas for easier treatment, she mentioned in passing that ringworm is also infectious to humans and said that the McCoys should wash their hands well after touching their pet. The couple seemed to perk up at this new information. Mrs. McCoy tried to ask Dr. Sally a question, but the buzz of the clippers muffled her soft southern drawl. Eventually, she was able to raise her voice just enough for Sally to hear her and turn off the clippers. In an almost embarrassed tone, Mrs. McCoy forced out the question: "Could this be the same problem that Henry has? Go ahead, Henry, show the doctor the area that's been botherin' you."

I heard the rattle of a belt buckle, then a very upset Dr. Sally yelling, "No, no, you need to show that to your own medical doctor!" Her usual confidence and composure had abandoned her. Now she was just as frazzled as I usually was. It gave me a little warm feeling inside when she shoved open the door, her face pale, shaking her head with frustration as she ran past me. Henry's ringworm lesion was in an area that should not have been exposed to anyone but his wife or a physician. The McCoys, however, must have figured they could kill two birds with one stone and save the cost of an extra office visit.

I asked Christie to help me finish treating Mr. Biscuits and sent the couple off to their family doctor. A few minutes later, Dr. Sally reappeared from the office area, where she had been hiding from the McCoys. Christie and I were in the process of cleaning up the exam room and sterilizing the Formica tabletop. Both of us were trying to hold back laughter, which caused our eyes to water and an occasional snort to escape. To our disbelief, Dr. Sally cracked a small smile, which meant the can was open. All three of us broke into a full-fledged roar that left us gulping for air.

The McCoys had managed to do what the rest of us could not—allow Dr. Sally to laugh at herself. From that day on, her time spent with us was a lot more enjoyable for everyone, including Dr. Sally, and ringworm cases took on a whole new meaning.

Animal Planet

In the mountainous areas of Colorado, you never know what you will run into or whom you might encounter next. Most people are not native to the area and have ended up in the mountains from other states or countries, and a certain percentage of these people are running from something, occasionally even the law. My years in this beautiful but rugged region have taught me that the snowcapped peaks can draw a rather eclectic crowd.

I have been lucky enough to meet many of these interesting characters during my years of practice, and these encounters always make for an interesting day. Some days I feel more like I am watching myself in a movie or dream than actually participating in the situation. One day in particular stands out in this category of surreal experiences.

It started out as a relatively routine summer morning, and most veterinarians like routine. We get enough surprises on a daily basis.

A feline needing dental work and a sheltie with a steak bone caught around its lower jaw got things started for the day—nothing to increase my blood pressure, but it was still early.

Christie caught me right after lunch to let me know that someone needed to go to the Anderson ranch to see a horse with a rope burn before the end of the day. My boss overheard the conversation while spaying a cat in the surgery room, but he kept his head down over the patient, concentrating on his work. Without looking up, he posed the inevitable question: "What are you doing this afternoon, Jeff?"

Since I easily interpreted this to mean "You will be making this call," I chuckled. "Sounds like I'm going to the Anderson place," I said, but I wondered why he so obviously didn't want to go. It was a long drive, yet I sensed that there was more to it than just the trip.

I had met Mr. Anderson only once. He had come into the clinic on a busy afternoon with a fecal sample from his horse. Worried that worms were causing the horse to lose weight, he demanded we run the fecal test immediately. He was about sixty-five years old, sporting bushy white hair and an unkempt white beard. Multicolored suspenders held up his soiled jeans, and his tattered flannel shirt had seen far better days. To run a stool sample, only a tiny amount of feces is required, yet he had brought in the entire bowel movement of the mature equine—in a pizza box. He then proudly displayed it in front of a waiting room full of pet owners. He seemed to find great humor in the turned-up noses and distressed faces of the clients seated around the shrinking space. I took it from him as quickly as possible, saving the thimbleful needed to run the test and throwing the rest away in the Dumpster outside, but not quickly enough to prevent the clinic from smelling like a barn. I had survived my first encounter with Mr. Anderson, but today it was time for round two.

Christie and I got the necessary directions and headed out, a little leery of what we might find. At a time when ranches in Colorado were quickly transforming into subdivisions, it was good to know that at least this one was still in operation. Our destination lay in one of the most beautiful regions of our practice, on a stunning high mountain plateau known as "the ridge." Surrounded by stunning peaks on all sides, it is forty miles wide by fifty miles long. The pass that gets you there tops out with a drop-jaw view of the entire area. A longtime resident of the ridge told me that when his great-grandfather had set up housekeeping on the plateau, the remnants of Ute tepees still dotted the landscape. Now only the ruins of cattle ranches are left, most of whose owners sold their water rights to Denver and its suburbs in the middle of the last century. Without water to irrigate the pastures, the remaining ranchers can keep very few cattle, and elk herds search out the sparse patches of grass.

The weather on the ridge can be harsh and unpredictable. Even in the summer, the temperature can drop thirty degrees in thirty minutes in the wake of a hailstorm. In the winter, the snow often comes down horizontally, thanks to raging winds, making it impossible even to see the hood of your car, let alone the edge of the road. The people and animals here are tough, independent, and not overly willing to accept strangers. The Andersons proved to be no exception.

The ranch included hundreds of acres, and the house sat strategically in the center of it, so there was an extremely long driveway. The weathered KEEP OUT sign beside the mailbox was the first clue to what was coming. Christie turned to me and raised a skeptical eyebrow. Glancing down at the directions, she mumbled, "Hope this is the right place." I nodded with equal skepticism as I headed the truck down the driveway. We drove for three long miles, which seemed like twenty, before spotting the main house. It was a classic ranch home, windblown, with a little white paint still holding on for dear life.

Our welcoming committee was a herd of some forty goats, which gathered around the truck, bleating and looking for food. I chased them away when they started eyeing the tires. There appeared to be no humans around except for a heavyset man and a grade school-age girl lapping at ice-cream cones on the front steps. They were either ignoring us or were just not aware of our presence, since they made no attempt to look up from their dessert. I told Christie to try to communicate with them while I gathered together my paper towels and antiseptic soap to clean up the injured horse. It always makes a better impression to appear a little prepared.

Just as I turned to start toward the house, I saw Christie coming back to the truck at a near run, terror in her eyes. She was pointing behind her as she came. I couldn't see what she was so worked up about at first. Then, as I moved just a little to see around Christie, the object that had rendered her speechless came into view. Tied to an old iron gate with a thin nylon rope was a full-grown African lion. It was surrounded by a pile of sun-bleached bones, presumably from livestock that didn't make it. The scene was so unreal that I had to blink my eyes several times to make sure it wasn't a movie—something between *Of Mice and Men* and *Out of Africa*. I was halfway expecting Meryl Streep to poke her head out the door at any moment to invite me in for pie. Unfortunately, she did not, and Christie had locked herself in the truck within seconds. It was up to me to let someone know we were here and find the patient.

I yelled to the pair on the steps. "Can you tell me where I could find Mr. Anderson?" The big man pointed into the house before returning to his disappearing cone, so I gave the kitty a wide berth and headed for the front door. Inside, I found a group of about ten motley cowboys sitting around a table covered with mounds of meat and potatoes. The group appeared to be a combination of every race and culture but all were tough-looking. I could have sworn I had seen a couple of them on the post office wall.

Mr. Anderson sat at the end with an authoritative posture, supervising the meal. His wife hurled bowls of food onto the table as she brought them in from the kitchen. She was a large gray-haired woman in her early sixties and didn't seem overly happy about her position as cook, waitress, and dishwasher. She occasionally scowled at the ranch hands, as if warning them not to stay at the table too long. Since it would take at least a three-hour drive to locate a McDonald's in either direction, the patrons here appeared to abide by her wishes.

I waited quietly for a few minutes, hoping someone would acknowledge my presence, and eventually Mr. Anderson raised his head just long enough to speak. "Horse is in the third barn, the tallest one. Someone will be out to help you as soon as we're done here." Then his eyes refocused on a large pitcher of gravy, and I realized I had been dismissed. A nod from Mrs. Anderson confirmed it, so I headed out to pry Christie out of the truck and find the horse.

The little girl, the large man, and the lion had lapsed into afternoon naps near the steps, allowing me to sneak by unnoticed. Clutching my supplies, I walked with Christie toward the tallest barn, one of many half-gone structures on the place. We ventured slowly into the building, which was well illuminated by the unintentional skylights in the old roof. Hoping not to find any more predators from the Dark Continent, we took every step cautiously, eventually catching a glimpse of the horse in a makeshift stall in the center of the barn. The animal was only about a year and a half old and obviously not well trained. He bucked and kicked in the stall, showing off for a new audience. I like to compare horses this age to teenagers, completely impossible to reason with. We decided to wait for help instead of risking bodily injury to ourselves. Christie and I sat down on a bale of hay to wait, figuring it couldn't be long—Mrs. Anderson would surely run them out of her house soon. We waited in silence while the young bay continued dancing in the stall, as if daring us to come in with him.

Suddenly, something fell from the rafters onto the floor in front of us. Startled, we both jumped to our feet and examined the object. It was some type of exotic bird, the likes of which neither of us had ever seen before. The avian creature was rather large, about eighteen inches long, with a bright red serrated cone on top of its head and a multicolored long, pointed beak. The rest of the bird was jet black. It definitely was not a normal resident of this area. Why was it lying dead on the floor in front of us? Squinting our eyes, we were able to make out the dark figures of similar creatures moving about in the rafters two stories up.

That was the end of the rope for Christie and me. We leaped into the pen with the young horse and, with the power of adrenaline driving us, grabbed the animal's halter. The horse seemed to sense that we were going to do the job no matter how much he objected, so he settled down and gave in to the treatment. I clipped the hair around the rope burn while Christie washed it up with antiseptic soap. Out of a need to leave the ranch as soon as possible, we worked together like a well-oiled machine. I covered the wound with ointment and scribbled out directions on a plastic container of antibiotic powder, leaving it behind on a bale of hay by the stall.

We gathered up our tools and made a break for the truck, again giving the house the wide berth it deserved. Our escape was almost complete when we stopped short in front of the pickup. At least fifteen goats were roaming about on the hood and fiberglass vet box in the back. The truck's paint was severely scratched, and the goats seemed to have done a week's worth of defecating on the windshield. At least another twenty-five goats, still on the ground, were trying to get onto the truck, but there wasn't any space left. Their sharp little hooves tore at the doors and fenders. Goats are extremely athletic, even the smallest ones. On my truck, they looked more like their Rocky Mountain cousins than the domestic variety they were. Normally, I would have been upset, but Christie and I wanted to leave so badly, we just chased the gang of caprine off and made tracks for civilization.

On returning to the clinic, I sent Mr. Anderson a bill that included a little extra to help cover truck repair. Needless to say, he was not happy and sent in a check that covered only the horse treatment. The envelope included a note indicating I might pick my parking spots more carefully in the future. The good news is that he never called back, and according to the neighbors, the horse recovered nicely. It's a good thing because we wouldn't have been able to afford any more auto-body work.

End of the Day

"Colicky horse in Sawmill Gulch—who wants to see it?" It was 4:55 on a Friday afternoon in mid-August, always a popular time for emergency calls to come in. This meant the lowest on the totem pole would be the one chosen for the job, and that meant me. We didn't recognize the last name, but the caller was to meet me at a nearby gas station, then lead me to the horse. Why they couldn't just give me directions bothered me a little, but I brushed it off as just a new client with a hard-to-find home.

Arriving at the station, I had no trouble picking out my guide. A twenty-year-old rust-scarred pickup with a large trailer hitch sat parked at the outskirts of the parking lot. One might have thought it was unoccupied except for the moth-eaten black cowboy hat barely showing above the steering wheel. I could just make out the face of a man under the hat. He had seen a lot of Colorado sun and probably wasn't nearly as old as he appeared. The hat nodded when I pulled in beside the vehicle, so I followed it back onto the road. A decent muffler was obviously not a priority for the driver, and the truck roared down the highway, belching black smoke. Even when I lost sight of him, I could still follow the noise and smell.

I had driven this section of road many times, but I still had a little trouble keeping up. Just when I thought I might actually lose him despite the noise and smoke, he turned off onto a dirt road. It was Sawmill Gulch Road, and I didn't remember ever having seen houses on it. A rough one-lane, it was really more of a path than a road. It was the only route into this region of national forest. I had been hiking in this area before and knew the parking lot that led to the trailhead was not much farther. The sick horse would probably be there, I reasoned, so maybe Marion and I would make it to that movie after all.

When the trailhead came into view, I spotted two horses tied to a horse trailer that had seen better days. The trailer's tires were completely bald, and paint was a distant memory. The horses had saddles and bridles on, but neither appeared to be ill. The hat jumped out of the truck in front of me and started for the steeds.

"Well," I said, "it looks like the animal is much better now. Which one was having the problems?"

The man pushed up his hat, exposing the big smile that was forming across his face. "These are our mounts; the one with colic is up the trail a ways," he began. "You'll have to put all the medication and equipment in these saddlebags so we can ride in. My wife is waiting with the sick one, so we'd better get going."

My first thought was, You've got to be kidding me. But someone had to take care of the poor animal, so I started transferring the supplies from my truck to the horse. The next thing I knew, I was actually riding a horse into the woods to treat another. I guess the owner just assumed that since I was a veterinarian, I should know how to ride a horse. If my classmates could only see me now, I thought, they would just shake their heads in wonder. Most of them would be leaving their clinics about then to get a good start on the weekend, maybe even heading to restaurants for a nice meal. A little food sounded pretty good at that moment.

As we rode, I began to get to know Mr. Ledger. He and his wife had come up from Denver for weekend trail riding. Their packhorse, Sue, had started to go down and began to roll, the classic signs of colic in a horse. Because the equine species is not capable of vomiting, intestinal blockages tend to be incredibly painful. They can be caused by anything from constipation to an intestinal torsion, the latter being the last thing I hoped to find.

After about fifteen minutes of riding, I was starting to get a little nervous. "How much farther?" I asked.

Mr. Ledger hesitated, then replied cautiously, "Ah, just around the bend. Won't be much farther now." I didn't entirely believe him, but what choice did I have? Besides, it was a beautiful evening for a ride. Forty-five minutes later, I began to hear noises ahead on the trail. In a small clearing was a sweaty, thrashing gray horse with a small middle-aged woman tugging on its lead rope to get it up. The animal wouldn't budge. Its abdomen was bloated, and its pain was so great that not even an atomic bomb would have been able to distract it.

I introduced myself to Mrs. Ledger, and she said, "Well, I hope you can do something quickly. I don't think she can last much longer, and neither can I." The two of them looked at me longingly, obviously wanting me to perform a miracle.

The horse lay on her right side at my feet, gasping for every breath. Her left eye turned up toward me with that "Please do something for me" look. Retrieving my stethoscope from the saddlebags,

I proceeded to examine the patient. Her heart rate was eighty beats per minute, way too high, and she had none of the normal intestinal sounds over the abdomen. My best shot at successful treatment was to reduce the pain so the intestines could relax, then get some laxative in her stomach.

After I injected Banamine into Sue's jugular vein and gave her a little sedative to calm her down, the distress seemed to melt away quickly, and soon Sue was able to get back onto her feet. She wasn't near 100 percent yet, but things were starting to look up. During the rectal exam, I was relieved not to find a torsion or intestinal twist, but there was a large amount of hard stool in Sue's cecum. This blockage was clearly the source of the problem. Being elbow-deep in a horse's rectum with the requisite shoulder-length latex glove is not very glamorous, yet it is still our best diagnostic tool for colic.

The Ledgers were elated to hear that there was no torsion. The horse would never have made it out of the forest if there had been. I got out the equine nasal gastric tube and passed it through her left nostril and into her stomach. Attaching the tube to the stomach pump, I pumped in the better part of a gallon of mineral oil, enough to loosen up almost anything! "Now we need to walk her for a bit to get the oil moving toward the blockage," I explained. The Ledgers nodded eagerly and immediately started walking the horse in circles.

After five minutes of walking, Sue started to pass gas and her bloating decreased. It was like the air being slowly let out of a balloon, except that this air was a little more pungent. As the gas passed, the horse felt continually better. A half hour later, the urge to lie down subsided, and it looked as if we would all make it out of the forest that night.

The Ledgers became more talkative at this point. "Doc, you did it! She's going to make it. Thank you so much," Mrs. Ledger said as tears of joy welled in her eyes. "We never thought we'd get anyone to come way back in here to treat her." I held back the urge to ask how many other veterinarians they had called before they got hold of me. Did they mention to the others that they'd be going on a one-hour trail ride each way?

The sun was beginning to go down over the mountain peaks as Mrs. Ledger wiggled herself up onto the now fully recovered equine. She took off down the trail bareback, with Mr. Ledger and me in tow. The next hour passed rather slowly, with many obstacles that wouldn't have seemed like such a big deal in full daylight. Now there were low branches to avoid and hard-to-see boulders in the trail. I was certain that every bend in the trail would open onto the parking lot. It was eight o'clock by the time we reached the trailhead, and a bigger-than-life moon had replaced the day's sun long before. As much as I would rather have been home with Marion by then, I had to admit it was a beautiful night for a ride.

We tied the horses to the trailer, where all three immediately commenced munching the hay that Mrs. Ledger put out for them, Sue included. I headed for the truck, and Mr. Ledger met me with his credit card held out. "I just can't thank you enough," he said. "I'm sorry we kept you out so late." I wrote up the bill and copied down his information.

Sliding into the truck, I waved my final good-byes, happy to be settling into the well-worn seat instead of the hard leather of the saddle. Pulling out of the parking lot, I rolled down my window and rested my arm on the ledge. I could just make out the silhouettes of the horses as they were being loaded back into the trailer for their ride home. The moon bathed the entire scene in soft light, giving it the appearance of a Western movie set.

I turned on the radio, flipping through stations until I found an old rock-and-roll station spinning a little Bob Seger. The crisp mountain air filled the cab of the pickup, diluting the smell of horse sweat that had permeated my clothes while I was treating Sue earlier. Once a war back on the pavement, my thoughts turned to Marion and some warmed-up supper. Like so many nights past, and even more that were to come, I couldn't wait to get home. I really hoped that the pager wouldn't go off that night. It would be awfully hard to face another call, but if one of my client's animals was in need, I would have to go. Fortunately, I have a wonderful, understanding wife, who is willing to put up with odd hours and late-night emergencies.

Afterword

The reality is that veterinary medicine is much more than just a career; it's a lifestyle. While its demands are sometimes frustrating, the rewards of being able to help animals and their owners can't be measured.

Veterinary medicine has also changed rapidly over the last twenty years. Mixed-animal practitioners, those who treat multiple species, are getting hard to find. Society's expectations, along with voluminous amounts of new medical information, dictate that we move toward more specialization. We now have veterinarians who work on only cats or dogs or birds. Some concentrate on exotics like snakes or lizards; others lean toward livestock. At this point, I devote nearly all my time to equine practice. I enjoy working with horses and their owners, but I often miss the humorous situations that mixed practice can present.

Another dramatic change in veterinary practice is that women have come to dominate the profession. My graduating class was composed of approximately 50 percent of each gender, but today male students are getting hard to find. Just over the last couple of years, women have even surpassed men in practice—quite a difference from what held true for most of the last century, when veterinary medicine was considered a "man's profession."

Sometimes in the middle of the night when I am called from my bed and no one else is on the road but elk, mountain lions, and an occasional state trooper, I wonder how good an idea my career choice was. Then a little girl with tears in her eyes thanks me for saving her pet, or a horse that appeared near death on my arrival is munching hay when I finally crawl back behind the wheel. These are the things that make veterinary practice more than just a job. It's these little rewards that enable one to overlook those times when an impatient client feels, in the midst of his concern, that his pet has the most urgent problem.

Veterinarians must be able to stand up to those animal owners who want them to do something that is against their better judgment, yet be there with a hug when a beloved pet dies. It's a profession that requires many hats, along with a good sense of humor, to keep one from going nuts. I've learned that veterinarians need to be capable of laughing not only at the situation but at ourselves as well.

The hours are long, the academic training is tough, and the pay isn't the best, but I can't think of many other professions that provide more variety on a daily basis or more personal satisfaction. Veterinary medicine is not for everyone. I always suggest that young people who believe they are interested in the profession spend a substantial amount of time working with a veterinarian to be sure that this is the right path for them.

I hope you have enjoyed riding along with me through my early years of veterinary practice—and we have only scratched the surface.